The

AIR
SELF-CARE
HANDBOOK

Breathe Easier and Protect Yourself from Pollution

MELISSA WROLSTAD

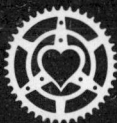

THE AIR SELF-CARE HANDBOOK

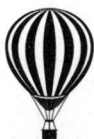

MELISSA WROLSTAD

Microcosm Publishing
Portland, OR | Cleveland, OH

The Air Self-Care Handbook
Breathe Easier and Protect Yourself from Pollution
Part of the DIY Series

© Melissa Wrolstad, 2026
This edition © Microcosm Publishing, 2026
First Edition, 3,000 copies, first published February 3, 2026
ISBN 9781648415517
This is Microcosm # 1042
Designed by Joe Biel and Sarah Koch
Edited by Lex Orgera

For a catalog, write or visit:

Microcosm Publishing
2752 N Williams Ave.
Portland, OR 97227

All the news from the misfits in print at www.Microcosm.Pub/Newsletter

Get more copies of this book at microcosm.pub/AirSelfCare

Did you know that you can buy our books directly from us at sliding scale rates? Support a small, independent publisher and pay less than Amazon's price at **www.Microcosm.Pub.**

To join the ranks of high-class stores that feature Microcosm titles, talk to your rep:
In the U.S. **COMO** (Atlantic), **ABRAHAM** (Midwest), sales@microcosm.pub (Texas, Oklahoma, Arkansas, Louisiana), **IMPRINT** (Pacific), **TURNAROUND** (UK, Africa, Middle East, Europe), **UTP/MANDA** (Canada), **NEWSOUTH** (Australia/New Zealand), **APD** (Asia), **HarperCollins** (India), and **FAIRE** in the gift trade.

Global labor conditions are bad, and our roots in industrial Cleveland in the 70s and 80s made us appreciate the need to treat workers right. Therefore, our books are MADE IN THE USA and printed on post-consumer paper.

LCCN 2025027836

Microcosm's workers and authors are paid solely from book sales. If you downloaded this book from some sketchy part of the Internet or picked up what appears to be a bootleg, please support our hardworking team by purchasing a copy directly from us and encouraging your communities to do the same. An MIT study revealed that AI inhibits humanity's critical thinking ability. Since critical thinking is one of our core values, we prohibit any use of our books to "train" generative artificial "intelligence" (AI) technologies, because seriously, WTF?

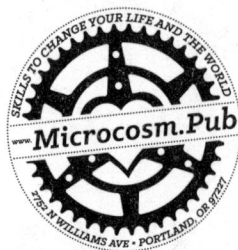

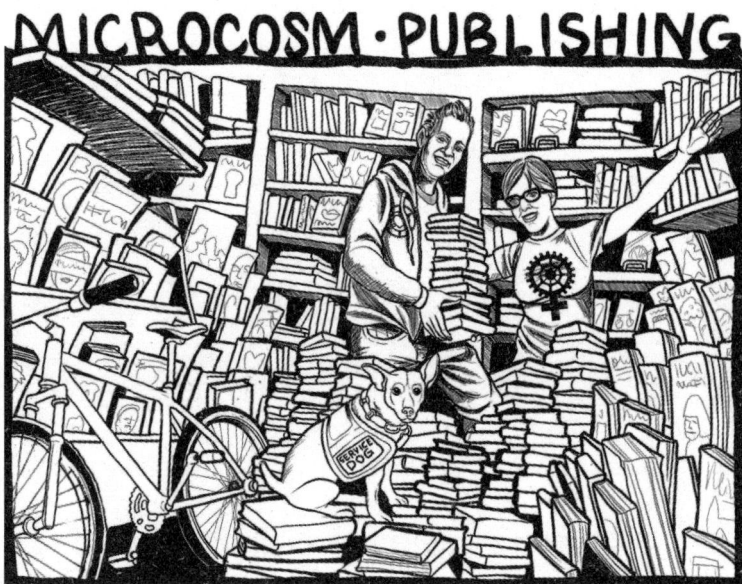

MICROCOSM · PUBLISHING

MICROCOSM PUBLISHING is Portland's most diversified publishing house and distributor, with a focus on the colorful, authentic, and empowering. Our books and zines have put your power in your hands since 1996, equipping readers to make positive changes in their lives and in the world around them. Microcosm emphasizes skill-building, showing hidden histories, and fostering creativity through challenging conventional publishing wisdom with books and bookettes about DIY skills, food, bicycling, gender, self-care, and social justice. What was once a distro and record label started by Joe Biel in a drafty bedroom was determined to be *Publishers Weekly*'s fastest-growing publisher of 2022 and #3 in 2023, and is now among the oldest independent publishing houses in Portland, OR, and Cleveland, OH. Biel is also the winner of PubWest's Innovator Award in 2024. We are a politically moderate, centrist publisher in a world that has inched to the right for the past 80 years.

♥ CONTENTS ♥

Dedicated to Mary Ann Schmitt, an outstanding lady.

INTRODUCTION

*D*ear Reader,

Air is what connects our lungs and, by way of the bloodstream, our hearts with the hearts of all living creatures on the planet.

As a person who had asthma as a kid and who still has trouble breathing when air quality is bad—this world can be a pretty scary place sometimes! Especially since there aren't a lot of people you can turn to that know much, if anything, about how to take care of themselves (or you) air-wise.

I've been fortunate enough to be educated on air quality through my work as an engineer and sustainability consultant. I'm frequently surprised at how air quality guidance these days is typically filled with piles of technical jargon and hidden away in textbooks and complex applications that feel inaccessible to anyone without a PhD in some sort of engineering design field. Plus, it's rarely taught in schools.

This has driven me to take time on my nights and weekends to sit down, digest current guidance on air quality, and write a book covering the basics for you. I've tried to format it in such a way that even if you consider yourself "math phobic" or one of the "I just don't get science" folks, you can feel like you've got the gist and are ready to rock on better air self-care by the end.

And what is air self-care? Pretty much exactly what it sounds like! It is guidance about air, air pollution, the impact air pollution has on us, and practices we can all follow to protect ourselves and our loved ones from the negative effects of air pollution.

Here is an overview of what this handbook covers:

- Chapters 1–3: Introduction to air, air quality, and air pollution basics
- Chapters 4–5: Air-related building design and interior air quality
- Chapters 6–7: Methods of air-pollution detection
- Chapter 8: Tackling indoor air quality issues
- Chapter 9: Preparing for unexpected poor air quality

The study of air and its impact on living creatures is vast and complex. In these chapters, I'm sticking to the fundamentals available per current science, and I am well aware that this book is by no means comprehensive. Over time, I hope air quality science will continue to develop, and I'll be able to update this handbook with inspiring new and refined guidance on how we can improve our air self-care practices.

As you work your way through each chapter, please remember that while this text is based in science and research, it is intended for educational and informational purposes and does not seek to provide professional medical advice. Always consult your doctor first about anything related to your health.

Before we start the book, I want to share that two days after I finished my first full-length draft, my home in upstate New York got hit hard by the first major Canadian wildfire smoke event of 2023. We got the eerie red sun for three days, and our view of far-off country hills slowly vanished until we almost couldn't even see the edge of our back porch. Our local wildlife was oddly hushed, and the air outside tasted of campfire smoke.

I had a moment while looking out onto this very surreal scene when I realized that the guidance I had compiled for this handbook had comprehensively prepared me to be safe and breathe easy during the entire event. With all the time and heart I'd spent over the past two years putting the book together, it was pretty emotional to see it all paying off, in my house.

The event gave me added perspective that I've used to polish off this handbook into a simple, practical guide that covers much, much more than how to handle wildfire smoke events. In Chapter 10, I'll circle back to this story and provide details on the specific air self-care steps our family followed to handle this wildfire smoke event, which will make a lot more sense once you've read Chapters 1–9!

🎈

And finally, to really emphasize how important knowledge on air and air quality is, did you know that air pollution kills an estimated seven million people worldwide every year?[1] This is:

- Over 2 times more than COVID deaths in 2020[2]
- Over 35 times more than war and conflicts in 2024[3]

1 World Health Organization, "Air pollution: Impact," accessed March 29, 2025, who.int/health-topics/air-pollution#tab=tab_2.
2 World Health Organization, "The true death toll of COVID-19," May 20, 2021, who.int/data/stories/the-true-death-toll-of-covid-19-estimating-global-excess-mortality.
3 Irene Mia, "The Armed Conflict Survey 2024: Editors Introduction," The International Institute for Strategic Studies, December 12, 2024, iiss.org/publications/armed-conflict-

- Over 1.75 million times more than fatal shark attacks in 2024[4]

And these are not dazzling or fast deaths in bright burning glory. These are oftentimes slow, painful, deaths from long-term diseases like lung cancer and heart disease. The World Health Organization (WHO) has provided research showing that almost all of the global population (99%) breathes air that exceeds WHO guideline limits for adequate air quality.[5] Per the 2020 report "State of Global Air/2020" published through a collaboration between the Health Effects Institute and the Institute for Health Metrics and Evaluation, poor air quality is "the fourth highest cause of death among all health risks, exceeded only by high blood pressure, tobacco use, and dietary risks."[6]

Truly, it is a dear wish of mine that the guidance in this book is helpful to you, your family, your friends, your pets, and *especially* anybody you know who understands what it's like to struggle to breathe.

Love, M

survey/2024/editors-introduction/.

4 Florida Museum of Natural History, "Yearly Worldwide Shark Attack Summary," accessed March 29, 2025, floridamuseum.ufl.edu/shark-attacks/yearly-worldwide-summary/.

5 World Health Organization, "Air pollution: Overview," accessed March 29, 2025, who.int/health-topics/air-pollution#tab_1.

6 Health Effects Institute, "State of Global Air 2020. Special Report," 2020, stateofglobalair.org/sites/default/files/documents/2022-09/soga-2020-report.pdf.

Air Fun Fact:

Scientists have recently estimated that our planet's air became oxygenated over two billion years ago, based on their study of the chemical composition of very, very, very old rocks! They theorize that there was a period of time, aptly named the Great Oxygenation Event (GOE), where cyanobacteria and other photosynthetic microorganisms stood up and said "this is our moment" and started cranking out boatloads of oxygen.[7]

7 Jennifer Chu, "Study pinpoints timing of oxygen's first appearance in Earth's atmosphere," Massachusetts Institute of Technology News, May 13, 2016, news.mit. edu/2016/oxygen-first-appearance-earth-atmosphere-0513.

I. AIR AND AIR POLLUTION

W hat is air exactly? We can't usually see it or hear it, but we can feel it on our skin when we flail our hands about or stand right next to a window fan.

As I'm sure you know, it's not a solid or a liquid—it's a gas!

And it's not a single gas; it is actually made up of about 78% nitrogen, 21% oxygen, and 1% other gases, including carbon dioxide and argon. It acts like the skin of our planet. NASA says air ends and space begins about 62 miles above the ground. For some added perspective, the International Space Station orbits Earth at about 200–250 miles above the planet.[8]

Science says our planet's air is divided into five layers: the troposphere, stratosphere, mesosphere, thermosphere, and exosphere. The only layer we're going to talk about in this book is the troposphere, since it's the one that we live and breathe in. (Unless you're some kind of wild-sports super skydiver, you're never going to be breathing air above the troposphere.)

---

8 National Aeronautics and Space Administration, "International Space Station," last updated May 23, 2023, nasa.gov/reference/international-space-station/.

Now, this air we live in has many talents, and one talent is that it can hold things.

When it holds an entire superjumbo plane with 500-plus passengers and their luggage, it's called "Wow, that airplane is flying!" When it holds water molecules, it's called things like humidity! Clouds! Rain! Snow! Fog! When air starts to hold things like soot and chemicals that come out of vehicle tailpipes or factory smokestacks, now we're talking air pollution.

You might think—why doesn't air make the right choice and say, "No, I won't hold that garbage for you"? But the truth of the matter is that air doesn't have a choice—it's a friend that carries what gets handed to it.

When we walk through air that is currently carrying around air pollution toxins, air doesn't set the pollution down kindly before it enters our mouths. It carries that air pollution right through our noses, mouths, throats, and right into our lungs.

We don't tend to hear about air pollution that much in the news unless it is extreme and gnarly looking. At the time of writing, these were some recent air pollution events in the news:

Beijing Olympics

Before the 2008 and 2022 Olympics, there was major media hubbub about air pollution in the host city Beijing, China. Before both events, China took drastic measures to prepare for the festivities, such as shutting down factories and significantly lowering the number of vehicles on the roads, thus reducing local air pollution and ensuring athletes would feel comfortable competing in the air quality conditions. According to the Centre for Research on

Energy and Clean Air, the levels of PM2.5 (fine dust, a common air pollutant that we'll talk about later in detail) dropped 56.1% from 2021 to 2022.[9]

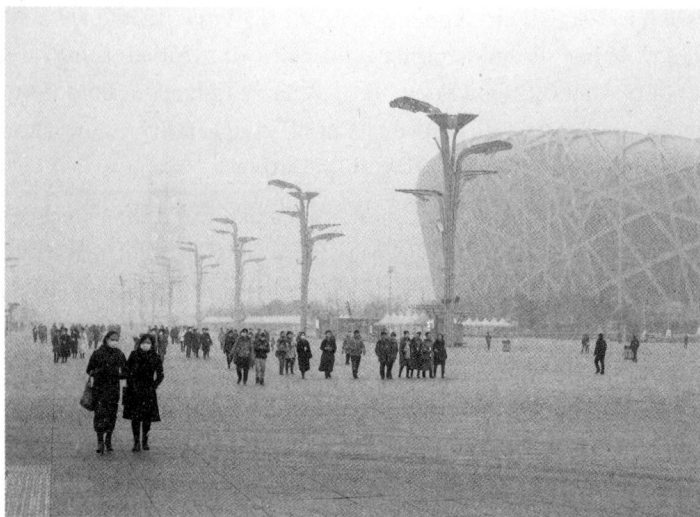

This photograph shows people walking past the Beijing National Stadium, also referred to as the Bird's Nest, built for the 2008 summer Olympics in Beijing, China. The air pollution is so dense that detail of the iconic stadium design is lost in the haze when viewed from a relatively close distance. You can also see a number of people wearing masks to protect themselves from breathing the pollution. Photo: © Xi Zhang

Australian Megafires

In 2019–2020, Australia experienced what the news titled "megafires" (i.e., major bushfires). These fires regularly made the news for many reasons, including the very poor air quality that contributed to substantial loss of both human and animal lives. The fires were so large they could be photographed from space.

---

9 Xinyi Shen, "Beijing Winter Olympic blue and China's long march against smog," Centre for Research on Energy and Clean Air, April 25, 2022, energyandcleanair.org/beijing-winter-olympic-blue-and-chinas-long-march-against-smog/.

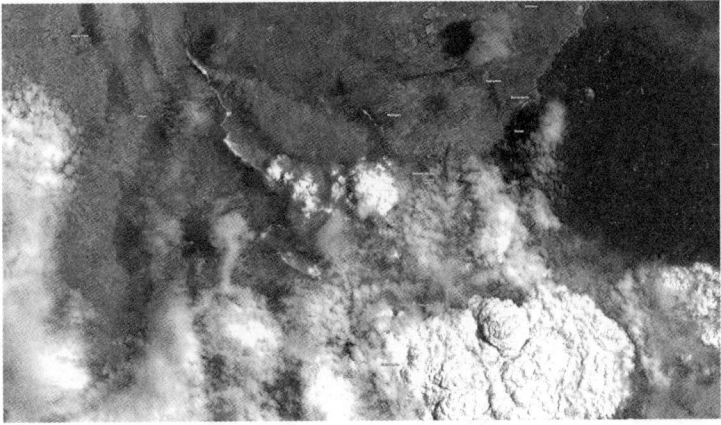

The Copernicus Sentinel satellite took this photograph of the 2019 Australian megafires. You can see the path of wildfire smoke billowing eastward across the continent. Photo: Copernicus Sentinel data (2019).

Air Quality Events in New York City

Wildfires in Canada and the United States have also been widespread in the early 2020s, causing the worst recorded air quality since 2006 when this type of data was first gathered.[10]

In June of 2023, wildfire smoke drifted from Canada over hundreds of miles of North America before totally blanketing New York City. You can watch the iconic city skyline totally disappear into wildfire smoke if you search online for "time lapse June 2023 wildfire smoke in New York City" videos.

---

10 Oliver Milman, "Air pollution in U.S. from wildfire smoke is worst in recent recorded history," *The Guardian*, June 8, 2023, theguardian.com/environment/2023/jun/08/air-quality-record-smoke-hazard-wildfire-worst-day-ever-canada-new-york.

New York City has had other significant air quality events, such as the 1953 smog that resulted in an estimated 170 or more deaths over a period of about ten days.[11]

The New York City Chrysler Building from the Empire State Building during a smog event in 1953.[12]

East Palestine Train Derailment

In early 2023 there was a train that derailed in East Palestine, Ohio that was full of toxic chemicals. The authorities decided that burning the chemicals was the safest way to dispose of them, and everyone within a one-by-two-mile area was required to evacuate

11 Robert K. Plumb, "DEATH RISE LAID TO '53 SMOG HERE; Report Says Daily Rate Was 17 to 26 Above Normal—All Ages Affected," *The New York Times*, July 3, 1961, nytimes.com/1961/07/03/archives/death-rise-laid-to53-smog-here-report-says-daily-rate-was-17-to-26.html?smid=url-share.
12 Albertin, Walter. "Smog obscures view of Chrysler Building from Empire State Building, New York City." Photograph. New York City, New York, 1953 November 20, accessed September 29, 2025. Library of Congress. loc.gov/pictures/item/95508508/

for multiple days due to dangerous, highly toxic fumes. There is still speculation on how far-ranging the damage was from this debacle on living creatures beyond the thousands of fish killed in the local water systems. Some believe animals were killed up to 10 miles away from the burn site[13] and there is still inconclusive information regarding the full impact of the event on local residents.

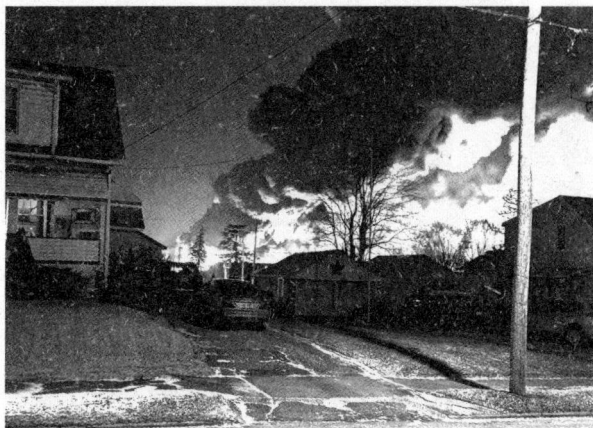

This photograph was taken from a person's front yard in a neighborhood close to the East Palestine train derailment site. Photo: Thunderlips

Now, the reality of things is that air pollution is much more rampant than these dramatic types of incidents that make the news, with pictures of highly visible, billowing plumes of black smoke or heavy smogs blanketing major city skylines.

Most air pollution is totally invisible to the naked eye!

Have you ever seen a truck on a highway belching horrid black fumes out its exhaust pipe? Within seconds, the black clouds of smoke fade into the air, but are they gone?

---

13 Nadine Grimley, "North Lima woman finds chickens dead Tuesday, questions chemical release from train," WKBN, February 7, 2023. wkbn.com/news/local-news/east-palestine-train-derailment/north-lima-woman-finds-chickens-dead-tuesday-questions-chemical-release-from-train/.

Nope! They've just dispersed to the point that you can't see them with the naked eye.

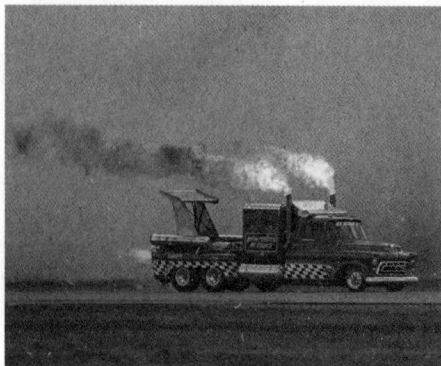

It's easy to forget that air pollution is being created around us except in those instances when we see spectacular displays of black smoke, like from this vintage truck "blasting the speed" down a highway with flames and black smoke on deliberate display. Photo: Y S

Some authorities will suggest that air pollution is "gone" once it has dispersed and you can't see it—but it is not gone. I will repeat— it is not gone. It has simply been spread around for more people and creatures on our beautiful blue-green planet to breathe.

Let's talk about some air quality situations that are direr—yes, direr—than the air quality situations that hit the news listed above, and yet, are totally invisible.

Evil Jeb

For visualization's sake, imagine a super villain named Evil Jebidiah, or Evil Jeb for short. Evil Jeb has no bones of good or justice in his body and hates kittens.

Now, imagine a room full of adorable mewing fuzzy kittens playing.

This is a photograph of a basket of adorable kittens with their entire lives of blissful, innocent, mayhem ahead of them. Like us, they depend on having access to clean air to thrive. Photo: The Lucky Neko

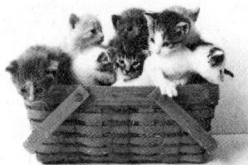

Evil Jeb has recently learned the coordinates of this room and wishes to eliminate the fluffballs posthaste. Here are things Evil Jeb could do to their air to accomplish his evil plans:

1. Suck the air out. No air means no oxygen for tiny kitten lungs to breathe, and they would all quickly suffocate.
2. Substitute the air (which is typically 20% oxygen) with air that is 10% oxygen or less. This would knock the little fluffballs out pretty quickly and, without having energy to eat, eventually they'd die.
3. Drop some potassium cyanide into a pan of hydrochloric acid to form hydrocyanic gas in the room. In this case, Evil Jeb would be eliminating the kittens with a form of capital punishment that is still legal in five U.S. states.[14]
4. Saturate the air with invisible and odorless viruses—literally waging biological warfare on the little dudes. The kittens, being ill-equipped for this type of warfare, would probably not make it.

May we never cross paths with Evil Jeb!

Now, if Evil Jeb's invisible air quality atrocities are too hypothetical for you, here is a real-world example of a serious air quality issue, also invisible to the naked eye, that resulted in many human casualties.

The Changcheng 361

In 2003, a Chinese submarine called the Changcheng 361 embarked on a planned lengthy training exercise with 70 naval crew members composed of both experienced and trainee cadets.[15] About ten days

---

14 Death Penalty Information Center, "Execution Method Descriptions," accessed March 29, 2025, deathpenaltyinfo.org/executions/methods-of-execution/description-of-each-method.
15 BBC News, "China sub victims 'suffocated'," May 5, 2003, news.bbc.co.uk/2/hi/asia-pacific/3001099.stm.

after leaving port, the submarine was discovered by some Chinese fishermen, eerily drifting near the surface of the water. According to reports from people that boarded the vessel to find out what was going on, all of the crew were dead and slumped over their stations. It was as though they were unaware of any impending problem at the time of their deaths. The most widely accepted theory of what happened on this submarine is that the diesel engines on the ship did not shut down correctly when the vessel submerged and quickly used up all available oxygen on the vessel—swiftly suffocating everyone.[16]

Most of us do not need to worry about imminently lethal air quality events because we don't do things like take rides on submarines. The invisible air pollution we're exposed to is milder and creates problems that hurt us over time.

Now, what exactly does regular exposure to moderate air pollution do to a human's (or pet's) respiratory system over time?

When we inhale, air travels through:

1. The insides of our noses
2. Our sinus cavities
3. Our mouth, including the teeth, tongue, hard palate, and soft palate
4. Our throat
5. Our lungs
6. Our bloodstream

16 *New York Times*, "Engine Trouble Suspected in China Submarine Disaster, Newspaper Says," accessed August 18, 2025, nytimes.com/2003/05/04/international/asia/engine-trouble-suspected-in-china-submarine-disaster.html. For those interested in the larger story that don't subscribe to the *New York Times*, there is a good Wikipedia article that has much of the same information, "Chinese submarine 361," accessed August 18, 2025, en.wikipedia.org/wiki/Chinese_submarine_361.

7. Organs in our body

8. Cells in our body

For so many reasons, we only want good stuff coming in! While the body does have certain ways of filtering air pollution out—like nose hairs, mucus, coughs, and sneezes—when there's a lot of it, it can get past these natural defenses and irritate and even damage interior surfaces of our bodies. It can get lodged in the lungs. Scarier yet, since the lungs are a direct passageway to the bloodstream, tiny, tiny air pollution particles can quickly enter directly into the bloodstream, circulate around the body, and do damage to organs like the brain and cells. A simple internet search will get you a long list of diseases and conditions that can either be caused or aggravated by air pollution. For those folks who have a valued daily skin ritual: air pollution is also bad for your skin, and can cause conditions like premature aging and skin irritation.[17]

So, what do we do then?

Well, first we start thinking about air and air quality on the regular.

To get us kicked off in this direction, I'd like to pose the following question: Do you pay as much attention to the 20,000-plus breaths you take into your body each day as you do to the food you eat 3–5 times per day?

To get your thought process cooking, let's take a glance at the words in our day-to-day vocabulary related to the air we breathe and the food we eat.

17 Ines Martic et. al, "Effects of Air Pollution of Cellular Senescence and Skin Aging," *Cells* 11, 14 (2022): 2220, doi.org/10.3390/cells11142220.

Please make a list of the "air" words that you use often in regular conversation. Here is a list I came up with during a quick sit-down: breath, breathe, air pollution, muggy, fresh, stuffy, wind, smoky, breezy, drafty, smelly, odor, hazy, foggy, whiff, atmosphere, and Pop Rocks (I love those little blasts of pressurized CO_2 on my tongue!).

Now, make a similar list of "food" words. Here is my list from a quick sit-down, or some of it! I needed to abbreviate my list in order to not take up too much prime real estate in this book:

- Food Varieties: croissant, tuna fish, broccoli, raspberries, chocolate, popcorn, peanut butter, pickles, pancakes, Pop Rocks
- Food Shopping: grocery store, farmer's market, patisseries, bodega, bakery
- Food Education: the food pyramid, the "food plate," food groups, nutritional education
- Food Diets: calorie counting, trans fats, plant-based, paleo, fruitarian, gluten-free
- Food Gone Bad: spoiled, rotten, curdled, moldy, overripe, expired, overcooked, burnt
- Restaurants: Michelin star, pizzerias, cafés, takeout, delis, restaurant critics, delivery
- Cooking and Baking Shows: Tons! There are even detective ones like *Crime Scene Kitchen*
- Holiday-Themed Cuisine: American Thanksgiving, birthday cake, St. Paddy's day milkshakes, UK Pancake Day, National Taco Day
- Organizations That Review and Approve Food: USFDA, Certified Organic, Certified Kosher

- Food Fun: flavors, monthly subscription boxes, taste testing, fondue fountain, cotton candy, space ice cream, Pop Rocks
- Food Adjectives: yummy, delicious, palate-cleansing, spicy, scrumdiddlyumptious
- Opportunities to Be Posh: French culinary school, seven courses, dessert spoon, Atlanta-based Poor Calvin's Absolute Fusion restaurant's lobster tail coated in Pop Rocks

My abbreviated "food" words list is *so much longer* than my "air" words list, and I'll bet yours is too! Mine probably also has three times as many references to Pop Rocks. (Candy that capitalizes on "air science" really tickles my funny bone.)

Getting back on track, why is it that we have so many more "food" words than "air" words when we breathe an awful lot more times a day than we eat?

My guess is it's because air is almost always invisible, and breathing happens (when you're lucky and have a healthy respiratory system) without much, if any, effort. Think about it—we can even breathe while we're sleeping. Really, unless you're having trouble breathing, it's easy to forget you're breathing at all. And so, we forget about air.

In the spirit of keeping air on our minds, let's start learning more about air, beginning with basics on outdoor air.

Air Fun Fact:

The longest satellite-tracked bird migration by air with no stops for food or rest is 8,435 miles from Alaska, United States of America to Tasmania, Australia, by a bird called the bar-tailed godwit! It took the little buddy—who was only five months old at the time—11 days. Way to go, champ! This epic journey is now commemorated in the Guiness Book of World Records.[18]

18 Aishwarya Khokle, "The record-breaking bird that flew from Alaska to Australia without stopping," Guinness World Records, January 3, 2023, guinnessworldrecords.com/news/2023/1/the-record-breaking-bird-that-flew-from-alaska-to-australia-731576.

II. OUTDOOR AIR BASICS

Outdoor air is a fancy term for "air outside."

Like, I wake up, walk out the front door, smile at the sunshine, and take in a deep breath to start the day. What's entering through my mouth and into my lungs is "outdoor air." Outdoor air includes all air that is outside of buildings and other human-made enclosed structures, including air in forests, air passing over cities, air over the ocean, air in open baseball stadiums, and the air that wild birds fly through.

To help you grasp and visualize the scope of worldwide outdoor air pollution—let me set you up with a mental picture of a smaller scale scenario that many of us have experienced firsthand:

It's a hot summer day, and the sun is so blazing that you've actually gotten organized enough to buy yourself some sunscreen even though it wasn't on sale. You pack your things, throw on some flip-flops, and head down to the local pool to cool off.

There are about fifty kids of a variety of ages already swimming in the pool when you arrive. You throw your stuff on a bench, plan your entry, and cannonball directly into the deep end. The cool water hits your skin all at once, and it's *glorious*. Just a little water gets up your nose, but it's worth it.

You paddle around for a couple minutes and then . . . somehow—maybe a little fairy whispers in your ear—you realize two kids have peed somewhere in the pool, and the old man treading water next to you is tooting regularly. (In this scenario, pool pee and toots constitute "water pollution.")

In the back of your mind, you *know* that somewhere there is a water filtration system sucking out old dirty water and replenishing it with fresh water—but how effective is the system? Is there pee or toot water currently on *your* skin? Was any of the water that just got up *your* nose . . . contaminated?

Thoughts start to unravel in your brain. You start asking even *more* questions like:

1. What level of kid pee, old-man toots, or other potential pool contamination like tiny baby poops is actually safe to swim in before you get some weird disease?
2. If the contaminated water in the pool isn't currently right next to you, how quickly will it disseminate to your section of the pool?
3. Should you get out immediately and shower five times?
4. Then, as you really start to get worked up . . . why don't the kids' parents tell their kids not to contaminate the communal pool water?
5. And finally—*Why don't people say when they've contaminated the water? 'Fess up!*—this water is getting in other people's mouths, ears, eyes, and belly buttons!

I hear you loud and clear my friend, I hear you loud and clear.

Keeping this scenario in your head, I want you to think of "outdoor air" as the water in the community pool. Like the water in the pool, air is scientifically also a fluid, and we share it with all other living outdoor creatures. (Science alert: Gases and liquids are both considered fluids and share properties such as the ability for their molecules to move around in constant random motion and bump into the walls of whatever container they are in. This is why the community pool analogy is especially apropos!)

Now, the good news is that there's a great deal more outdoor air around us than water in that community pool to help disperse contaminants. For example, an old-man toot does a lot less damage at the scale of "all outdoor air" than in the significantly smaller community pool.

That said, given that air is much less dense than water, pollutants can spread much faster. For example, in July 2021, New York City experienced the worst air quality it had seen since 2006 due to wildfires on the west coast of the continental United States, over 3,000 miles away.[19] As a resident of New York City at the time, I can say that it smelled strongly of wildfire smoke, and we largely stayed indoors for a couple days until the wildfire smoke passed. Then, just two years later in June 2023, the wildfire smoke traveling south from Canada was so severe that it blew the 2021 New York City air pollution levels out of the water. This wildfire smoke pollution from the north was spotted as far south as Alabama, over 1,000 miles away![20]

19 Hollie Silverman et al, "Western wildfire smoke is contributing to New York City's worst air quality in 15 years," CNN, July 21, 2021, edition.cnn.com/2021/07/21/weather/us-western-wildfires-wednesday/index.html.
20 Elizabeth Wolfe and Joe Sutton, "Smoke from hundreds of Canadian wildfires blankets northern U.S. cities with air pollution," CNN, July 25, 2023, cnn.com/2023/07/25/weather/canadian-wildfire-us-air-pollution/index.html.

In addition to wildfires, here are some other major player air polluters that you would not find in the community pool:

- Industrial Polluters
  - Large-scale agricultural animal raising (specifically the animal toots and burps)
  - Large-scale farming that includes spraying pesticides, herbicides, and/or fertilizers
  - Mining endeavors (specifically in blasting, excavating, and transport that can release particulate matter, heavy metals, and greenhouse gases into the air—ever heard of the black lung?)
  - Power plants and factories (specifically the emissions resulting from burning fossil fuels)
  - Refrigerants in cooling and refrigeration systems (largely responsible for the hole in the ozone layer)
- Natural Polluters
  - Dust storms—keep in mind, human-made practices such as deforestation can make dust storms more likely to happen
  - Flowering plants—while not considered air pollution by everyone, pollen is considered a highly annoying form of air pollution by many allergy sufferers
  - Volcanoes! These can really mess with air quality over large swaths of the planet when they belch large amounts of particulate matter, sulfur dioxide (a main instigator in acid rain), and other pollutants into the air.
- People Polluters
  - Airplane and space travel release particulate matter and emissions, like nitrogen oxide, from burning fossil fuels.

- o   Fireworks—one of my favorites, but so much smoke! (particulate matter)
- o   Food waste, both from regular folks like us and from the systems that bring us food. Did you know that food waste results in over half of landfill methane emissions?[21] Methane can lead to ozone, a serious air pollutant, at ground level.[22]
- o   Vehicle traffic like tailpipe emissions as well as tire and brake pollutants
- o   Wood and oil burning for home heating and cooking—again, particulate matter from burning fossil fuels

Taking a look at this list it can all feel a bit overwhelming, since most of us don't have control over many of the outdoor air polluters above (*especially* the volcanoes). If you're experiencing any frustration at this point in time or in the future and want to make a difference, I encourage you to skip to Appendix I entitled: "For Those Who Are Unsatisfied with the Status Quo" for some ideas on where to focus your energy.

Before we get into a list of actions we can take to protect ourselves and our loved ones from outdoor air pollution, I'd like to take the liberty to answer a few interesting questions.

---

21 United States Environmental Protection Agency, "Quantifying Methane Emissions from Landfilled Food Waste," last updated March 20, 2025. epa.gov/land-research/ quantifying-methane-emissions-landfilled-food-waste.
22 Erin E. McDuffie et al, "The social cost of ozone-related mortality impacts from methane emissions," *Earth's Future*, 11, 9 (2023), doi.org/10.1029/2023EF003853.

Question #1: Should I move to the boonies, to a place where air is *always* pristine?

A: There are general areas of the world where air is, on average, less polluted than in other areas. But, given the way air pollution travels, there is actually no location on the planet that is completely free of air pollution. I'll say that one more time so it sinks in: *There is no place on Earth that is 100 percent safe from air pollution.* As mentioned before, pollution from the wildfires in the west of the United States traveled across the country, over 3,000 miles west to east, and then a couple of years later, over 1,000 miles north to south—so, the *entire* continental United States is out.

Next, let's take a look at Antarctica.[23] You might initially think, "Wow, a place unaffected by humans because almost no knuckleheads live there!" And yet, the largest ozone layer hole, caused by refrigerants and similar air pollutants generated in other parts of the world, has resided primarily over Antarctica. Scientists have also identified lead pollution in Antarctic ice cores dating back to the industrial revolution that could have only traveled all the way to the South Pole via air.[24] *Again*, there is *no* location on the planet that is 100 percent air pollution-free.

Question #2: Can we just install a giant outdoor air purifier to clean the local air?

A: Unlikely. As of 2025, the technology to purify outdoor air at a large scale is still in a relatively fledgling state.

Let's say your city was able to afford and install one of the lovely new Smog Free Towers by Dutch artist Daan Roosegaarde that can treat up to 30,000 cubic meters (about 7.9 million gallons)

23 Daniel T. Gieseke, "Antarctic Pollution Issues," *International Pollution Issues*, December 2014, intlpollution.commons.gc.cuny.edu/antarctic-pollution-issues/.

24 J.R. McConnell et al, "Antarctic-wide array of high-resolution ice core records reveals pervasive lead pollution began in 1889 and persists today," *Sci* Rep 4, 5848 (2014), doi.org/10.1038/srep05848.

of air per hour.[25] Sounds like a lot of air! How long would it take to treat all of the air in your city? (First, fun sidebar: Daan the Dutch artist's studio transforms the collected smog particles from these towers into jewelry called Smog Free Rings.[26] I want one!)

Now, we need to make a few assumptions to estimate a timeframe:

- Assumption 1: This tower could actually process all of the air in your city. Air towers are a bit like fans—they can only push and pull air within a certain distance of their base. However, we will disregard science and assume this tower can access all city air.
- Assumption 2: An average city size of 355 square miles.[27]
- Assumption 3: A city height of 0.62 miles. This is about the height of an average low cloud like a cumulus cloud,[28] which is just a bit higher than the tallest building in the world (0.51 miles tall).[29]

These assumptions make the total city air volume:

$$355 \text{ square miles} \times 0.62 \text{ miles} = 220.1 \text{ cubic miles}$$

The estimated number of hours to clean the city's air one time with this device is:

$$\frac{220.1 \text{ cubic miles}}{\sim 7.9 \text{ million cubic gallons/hour}} = 30{,}675{,}000 \text{ hours} = 3{,}502 \text{ years}$$

That's a long time!

25 Studio Roosegaarde, "Smog Free Tower," accessed March 29, 2025, studioroosegaarde. net/project/smog-free-tower.
26 Studio Roosegaarde, "Smog Free Ring," accessed March 29, 2025, studioroosegaarde. net/project/smog-free-ring.
27 Ben Schulman and Xiaoran Li, "Population Ain't Nothing But a Number: Standardizing the Size of the Great American City," BELT Magazine, August 12, 2024, beltmag. com/population-aint-nothing-number-standardizing-size-great-american-city/.
28 National Oceanic and Atmospheric Administration, "The Four Core Types of Clouds," last updated March 28, 2023, noaa.gov/jetstream/clouds/four-core-types-of-clouds.
29 Encyclopaedia Britannica, "Tallest buildings in the world," last updated January 30, 2024, britannica.com/topic/tallest-buildings-in-the-world-2226971.

Question #3: Can't we just throw all air polluters in jail for contaminating our shared air?

A: Money and politics immediately get involved in this discussion. The internet is a treasure trove of battles fought so that you can have cleaner air to breathe. Some have been won and some have been lost. Unsurprisingly, there are very few, if any, people that have actually gone to jail for contaminating our air (and believe me, there have been some major contaminators). Some companies have had to adjust their processes, others have received fines for not complying, some are still in litigation, and some are still getting away with their air polluting shenanigans. The U.S. EPA (Environmental Protection Agency) has posted a list of successful resolutions regarding civil cases and settlements related to the Clean Air Act[30] (passed in 1970 with revisions in 1977 and 1990) on their website.[31] You will see that major cases are still being resolved in the 2020s!

After certain wins, you may have seen updates to vehicles over the years, resulting in fewer toxic emissions. The U.S. EPA has kept fascinating data[32] on trends since the 1970s, demonstrating the progress of the automotive industry in regards to increased fuel economy and the subsequent decrease in air pollution.

Separately, to comically complicate matters, many of us put certain forms of air pollution directly into our lungs with activities such as smoking and vaping. Should we throw ourselves in jail?

---

30 United States Environmental Protection Agency, "Clean Air Act Requirements and History," last updated August 6, 2024, epa.gov/clean-air-act-overview/clean-air-act-requirements-and-history.

31 United States Environmental Protection Agency, "Civil and Cleanup Enforcement Cases and Settlements," last updated March 12, 2025, epa.gov/enforcement/civil-and-cleanup-enforcement-cases-and-settlements.

32 United States Environmental Protection Agency, "Highlights of the Automotive Trends Report," last updated November 25, 2024, epa.gov/automotive-trends/highlights-automotive-trends-report.

With those fun questions out of the way, let's talk about air self-care when we're hanging out in outdoor air!

Outdoor Air Self-Care includes two main practices:
1. Regularly checking the local daily outdoor air quality
2. Familiarizing yourself with typical outdoor air quality patterns in places where you often spend time outside

Just two things—totally doable! Let's get into some more detail.

Regularly Check the Local Daily Outdoor Air Quality

A surprising number of us are fortunate enough to live relatively close to a station that measures outdoor air pollution for our region. There are websites that post data from these stations and have a similar feel to websites where you check the daily weather. In fact, some major weather reporting platforms are starting to incorporate air quality information into their online user interfaces.

If you're not sure where to start, head to the internet and search for the term "air quality index" (AQI) and fill in the location you're interested in. (A couple commonly used websites of this sort are AirNow.gov and IQAir.com.) The website will give you an AQI number that's between zero and infinity, where zero signifies air with zero air pollutants (of the pollutants that are monitored), and infinity is air with infinite air pollutants (h-yikes!). Since air typically has an AQI of less than 500, most dashboards that show the AQI will top out at 500 (not infinity). For more detail on how the AQI is calculated, please check out Appendix III: AQI 101.

What's nice about AQI is that it comes color-coded, so all you need to know is the color scheme to make informed air self-care decisions. A high-level summary of the colors is: green is good, yellow is okay, orange is not great, red is bad, purple is very bad, and maroon is very *very* bad. These classifications assume that the people and pets in question have healthy respiratory systems. Folks with serious breathing sensitivities may want to adjust this scale and consider yellow as "not great," orange as "bad," and so on.

Remember the community pool story? Here are some pool scenarios that correspond metaphorically with the AQI color scheme to help you make sense of the color scale:

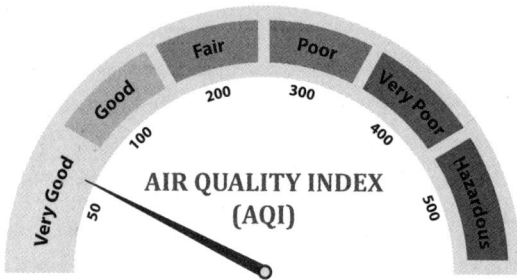

Fair Poor

Good 200 300 Very Poor

100 400

Very Good **AIR QUALITY INDEX** Hazardous

50 **(AQI)** 500

Green *(Very Good)*
Zero to one kids peed. For those of us that love pristine pool water, it's tough to realize that the water may just never be perfectly pristine. There's always a little pee in the pool, and it's probably not dangerous.[33] General research guidance says it's safe and you're good to continue doing what you do!

Yellow *(Good)*
One to two kids peed. It's not great, but keep in mind the pee gets diluted by a whole lot of other community pool water, and if you

---

33 Cleveland Clinic, "'Urine' for Some Bad News: Peeing in a Pool Isn't a Good Idea," June 22, 2023, health.clevelandclinic.org/should-you-really-pee-in-the-swimming-pool/.

don't think about it too much, you can relax and enjoy yourself because technically it's not dangerous unless you have specific sensitivities to pee on your skin or in your mouth . . .

Orange *(Fair)*

Three to five kids peed in quick succession, and things are getting legitimately gross in portions of the pool. At this point, you can't really avoid getting out of the pool unscathed. If you're *really* set on swimming, robust healthy people will still fare well and recover beautifully—but do you really want to do that to yourself?

Red *(Poor)*

Someone definitely pooped. Maybe that cute kid with all the curls and that peculiarly satisfied smile. In reality, most pool guests will survive just fine in this situation, but pretty much everyone is getting the eff out for very good reasons, and there's definitely a chance that some folks with weaker constitutions may get sick from exposure to the "pollution." Seriously, it's recommended that you get out and come swim another day.

Purple *(Very Poor)*

Mr. Whosit's Discount Construction team didn't check before doing some major construction right next to the pool. Some pipes and concrete were impacted, and now there's a sewer-leak situation seeping into the water. They say it's not a *gushing* leak, but holy smokes, the pool is also *not* the place to be. A competent pool management staff will get everyone out of the pool immediately and shut it down until the problem is fixed.

Maroon *(Hazardous)*

Think of a *bad situation*. Perhaps there's a massively contagious stomach flu ripping through everyone swimming in the pool, and things start to get *real* dicey. You suddenly find contagious vomit floating past your elbow—time to go! Good luck, my friend, because in this situation, it's unlikely even those of us with the most robust immune systems will come out unscathed.

You're welcome.

If you're not sure how to use AQI to inform your plans for the day, try making decisions like how you might make decisions based on the weather report. Here's my personal guide that compares AQI to weather situations that would similarly impact my plans (as someone who likes to be inside when there's inclement weather):

AQI Color	Forecast Weather
Green	Beautiful sunny day, perfect temperature—get out and do all the outside things.
Yellow	A bit icky out. Maybe some misty rain. Fine to do outdoor events, but not ideal.
Orange	Cold pouring rain all day. A good day to stay indoors if possible.
Red	Raging thunderstorms. Will definitely make plans to stay inside, and take a raincheck on any outdoor plans.
Purple/Maroon	Severe weather alerts. Time to batten down the hatches!

I hope this gives you some idea of how to assess your plans for the day depending on the outdoor AQI reading!

Now let's move onto the next aspect of outdoor air self-care.

Familiarize Yourself with Typical Outdoor Air Quality Patterns

While checking the AQI is very handy when you're making plans for the day, what happens when you're trying to plan for an event that is further into the future?

Well, air quality often ebbs and flows in regular patterns like the tides, fashion, fads, and fortune. These patterns can allow you to make educated predictions on air quality. Here are some examples of patterns that you can familiarize yourself with.

Seasonal Ebbs and Flows

Air quality can vary from spring to summer to fall to winter. Depending on where you are located in the world, there may be season-specific patterns of weather and human activity that can help you predict air pollution patterns in your area.

In many parts of the world, you can visit air quality websites and look at annual air quality data from the previous five or so years to see if there are any trends in your area. I've included some examples below of what it is possible to find after doing some detective work.

Example 1: London, England

One of the primary air pollutants that is tracked in outdoor air is PM2.5, also called "fine dust" (which we'll learn more about in the next chapter, along with other major air pollutants). If you look at annual PM2.5 levels in London, England, you will see that levels are typically significantly worse than normal in parts of March and/or April. Why is this?

It turns out farmers outside of London typically spray their crops in the spring, which releases contaminants that remain suspended in the air for the local population to breathe.

When your English gal pal is training for a marathon next spring, you can tell her, "Hey mate, check the outdoor AQI before training outside in March and April because the farms might be crop spraying, cheers!"

Example 2: United States of America

The United States of America's national Fourth of July holiday is frequently celebrated by epic fireworks displays in each town. When the fireworks are particularly spectacular and there are many towns in the region putting on displays on the same night, this can result in a significant temporary spike in PM2.5 levels.

When your American buddy is training for his first half-marathon over the summer, you might say to him, "Hey bro, you might want to wait to train outside until a day or so after the rad July Fourth fireworks displays are over. Catch you on the flip side!"

Example 3: Delhi, India

If you look up annual PM2.5 levels in Delhi, you will see that levels are typically significantly worse than normal in November, December, and January. It turns out that farmers burn crop waste (also called stubble burning) around November. Many people also start heating their homes around that time with fuels that create air pollution. In addition to this, Delhi deals with winter weather events that trap polluted air in one location instead of letting it disperse so it can get diluted (we'll talk more about these weather events soon). A triple whammy!

When your Indian pen pal is training for their first triathlon over the winter months, you might say, "Dear pen pal, I hope this letter finds you in good spirits. I've heard that AQI can be poor during the winter months, and I'm concerned about you training outside at that time. Please do the needful!"

Daily Ebbs and Flows

Air quality can also vary by time of day. It may be more difficult to access hourly AQI data than daily data. You can contact your local air testing station operator to see what they can make available to you. Here are some examples of daily air quality fluctuations that might occur near you.

Example 1: Ozone Smog

Summertime in New York City, Los Angeles, and other cities with regular traffic jams can see particularly high levels of ozone smog.

Ozone smog is often created when car exhaust and other types of smoke exhaust are graced by sunlight. The word smog was created in the early twentieth century to describe a mix of smoke and fog—creative, right?[34] Or sad, since apparently this type of air pollution was such a common occurrence around coal-burning industrial plants that they needed a new word!

Interestingly enough, once the sun goes down, the ozone smog dissipates, and you'll see that air quality improves until the sun comes out again.

When your neighbor is training for the local 5K fundraiser race over the summer in your city with lots of traffic, you might want to holler, "Hey neighbor, try training outside early in the morning or after the sun's gone down to avoid smog. See ya later alligator!"

---

[34] Hilary Costa et al, "Smog," National Geographic, last updated October 1, 2024, education.nationalgeographic.org/resource/smog.

Example 2: PM2.5 (Fine Dust)

A study was conducted in 2018 to determine when PM2.5 levels are the lowest during a typical day.[35] It turns out, after collecting and analyzing data from North America, Europe, and East Asia, the highest levels of PM2.5 occurred typically around midnight and 7 a.m. to 1 a.m., while the lowest levels per day were typically between 3 p.m. and 5 p.m.! Of course, this is averaged across the entire northern atmosphere, so this pattern may not strictly be the case in any specific area in the northern hemisphere.

If it *is* the case in your area, next time you see that same neighbor training for a run, you might yell, "Hey neighbor, actually, why don't you check the AQI before training in the morning and postpone until later in the day if it's bad? After a while, crocodile!"

Weather-Influenced Ebbs and Flows

Air quality can also vary based on the weather. For example, some weather systems can trap air pollution in one location so that it concentrates and gets worse, whereas other weather systems can dilute pollution or even clean it out of the air! If you are in a location experiencing poor air quality, keep an eye on the weather to predict how air quality might change in the near future. Below are some examples of how weather can affect air quality.

Wind

I had a professor in college that used to always say, "The solution to pollution is dilution." When it comes to air, wind is the primary pollution dilution solution since it can quickly mix more pristine air with the polluted air to create *less* polluted air. Keep in mind, wind isn't always the good guy. Wind can also carry air pollutants from polluted areas into less polluted areas, like in our examples of

35 Max I. Manning et al, "Diurnal Patterns in Global Fine Particulate Matter Concentration," Environmental Science & Technology Letters 5, 11 (2018): 687-691, doi. org/10.1021/acs.estlett.8b00573.

wildfire smoke traveling across the United States and the example of lead making it all the way to Antarctica.

Rain

Rain serves many purposes, like replenishing our water supplies, watering crops, and inspiring music like "Singing in the Rain" and Rihanna's "Umbrella." Another purpose it serves is to wash air pollution out of the air. It's like a giant happy air-washing machine. The sweet little raindrops take ahold of crap in the air, and drag it down to the ground so that we don't breathe it in anymore. However, watch out—when toxins in the air include sulfur dioxide and nitrogen oxides, this may mean acid rain falling on everybody below.

Lightning

Research based on data collected by some very brave pilots flying around massive storm clouds in 2012[36] has shown that lightning also cleans air![37] It produces hydroxyl radicals (OH) which are oxidizers (like dish detergents, laundry detergents, and bleaches) that can clean out air pollutants. You can think of lightning as a bleach detergent thrown into the giant happy air-washing machine (a.k.a. rain) to get the air squeaky clean!

Hot, Sunny Days

Direct sun and heat can cause chemical pollution in the air to react and result in something we'll call "air quality gnarliness," like the ozone smog from vehicle traffic we just talked about.

36 National Oceanic and Atmospheric Administration Air Resources Laboratory, "Lightning Produces Molecules that Clean Greenhouse Gases from the Atmosphere," accessed March 29, 2025, arl.noaa.gov/news-pubs/arl-news-stories/lightning-produces-molecules-that-clean-greenhouse-gases-from-the-atmosphere.
37 W. H. Brune et al, "Extreme oxidant amounts produced by lightning in storm clouds," *Science* 372, issue 6543, 711-715 (2021), doi.org/10.1126/science.abg0492.

Heat Domes

A heat dome occurs when hot air gets trapped over land, like a cruise liner that's gotten stuck on a giant sand dune. This "dome" holds hot air in one place, causing oftentimes dangerous heat situations that can span over days or even weeks. Aside from the heat dangers of this situation, air pollution can get trapped and continue to build up inside the heat dome (like germs or bad moods building up on the grounded cruise liner). When the heat dome lifts, the built-up air pollution can finally disperse.

Cold Weather Inversions

These inversions occur when hot air sits over cold air and holds it in place, like when you find a hairy spider on your side table and you put an upside down whiskey glass over it to keep it contained until you decide you're brave enough to take it outside. Any time air is held in place for a period of time, there is an opportunity for air pollutants from local air polluters to build up. Just like with the heat dome—air pollution can't disperse until the cold weather inversion lifts. These inversions are what trap the winter pollution in Delhi, India!

Given what you know now about weather, you can tell your aunt who's training for a breast cancer walk over the summer, "Hey Auntie! When you're training and see there's a heat dome, a really hot and sunny day, or wind blowing in from the direction of the super-dirty power plant, please do your walking inside at the mall with the great air conditioning. Lots of love!"

Now that we've spent some quality time learning about outdoor air, it's time to take a look at what happens when outdoor air strolls in through the front door.

Air Fun Fact

Air houses massive parts of our planet's water cycle. Clouds that carry rain, snow, and sleet across the sky are born and live in the air. One study—based on about a decade's worth of satellite pictures of Earth—estimated that at any time, about 67% of the Earth is covered in clouds, with most resting over our oceans.[38] These clouds are constantly moving water through the air and across the globe to keep us humans and the world's plants and animals properly hydrated.

38 National Aeronautics and Space Administration Earth Observatory, "Cloudy Earth," accessed March 29, 2025, earthobservatory.nasa.gov/images/85843/cloudy-earth.

III. INDOOR AIR BASICS

*A*ir is just the same old air anywhere, right?

Nope!

There are some very different things to consider when it comes to indoor air quality than what we talked about with outdoor air quality—so many things, in fact, that indoor air is what most of the rest of this handbook is about! To illustrate the difference, time for another story:

Your kid sister Sally won a couple of goldfish at the town fair, and she has nowhere to put them.

Mom says you can only keep them if they have a place to live, and Sally looks at you with puppy dog eyes that could sink a warship. Long story short, the two of you head to the local pet store to pick up a fish tank. The clerk tries to sell you things like a filter and some equipment to aerate the tank. At this point in your life, you couldn't care *less* about fish tank maintenance. You spent almost all of your allowance at the fair, and you're only prepared to fund the tank and some meager fish food.

You and Sally arrive home from the pet store, fill the aquarium with water, throw the fish in with some fish food and hope for the best.

Five weeks later, the big question is . . . *Are the fish in the aquarium still alive and thriving?*

Let's say Sally did a good job feeding them regularly, so they haven't gone hungry. But their living situation is missing an aerator, which would have brought new oxygen into the tank for the fish to "breathe." Their tank is *also* missing a filter to remove the literal fish crap and other nasties from their water. Five weeks in, you've probably got a relatively foul water situation going on, with questionable oxygen levels.

Has Sally gotten lucky and her fish from the fair are excellent at thriving in toxic wasteland conditions? Or have her fish given up the ghost and made a journey to their final resting place, starting at the family toilet? The fact that this is the current question on the table doesn't bode well for the fish. If you had bought the aerator and the filter, there might be a completely different question on the table at this point like, "Are we ready to add a sweet little snail who will be cute *and* help keep the tank clean?"

Why are we talking about Sally's aquarium?

Well, when we're looking at indoor air, it's basically outdoor air that has been contained in a fixed space—like water that's been poured into a tank.

Before you and Sally put that water in that tank, it was part of a larger ecosystem or municipal water treatment system with processes to care for that water. However, once you and Sally poured it into the tank, the larger ecosystem or municipal water treatment system could no longer care for the water, and the responsibility for care passed over to the two of you. Since you decided to add pet fish who would obviously be eating, pooping, and playing around in the water, love and care were required to maintain healthy water quality for them to live in.

Similarly, when air is outside, the wind and storms help dilute air pollution and clean out the nasties. When this air is "poured" into an enclosed room, outdoor wind and storms are no longer present to help clean the air. Love and care is now required to maintain the quality of the air, *especially* since there are people and pets living their lives in it! Just like in a well-tended fish aquarium, a well-tended room will have a method to facilitate new oxygen entering into the room and a way to get nasties (in this case, air pollution) out.

For the sake of this example, our buildings and homes can be thought of as stacks of aquariums of air, each one needing regular care. Throughout the rest of this handbook, I will sometimes refer to rooms as "air aquariums" that we need to tend to as part of our air self-care practices.

The United States EPA studies of human exposure to air pollutants indicate that indoor levels of pollutants may be two to five times—and occasionally more than one hundred times—higher than outdoor levels![39] The EPA also reports that "most people spend about 90 percent of their time indoors."[40] Not quite as high as Sally's pet fish who spend 100 percent of their time in their aquariums, but not too far off.

---

39 United States Environmental Protection Agency, "Why Indoor Air Quality is Important to Schools," last updated November 12, 2024, epa.gov/iaq-schools/why-indoor-air-quality-important-schools.
40 United States Environmental Protection Agency, "Indoor Air Quality," last updated July 8, 2024, epa.gov/report-environment/indoor-air-quality.

To put some icing on this unsavory cake, consider this quote found on the EPA website at the time of writing: "EPA does not regulate indoor air, but we do offer assistance in protecting your indoor air quality."[41] I wonder if they make house calls! (Just kidding, they don't. They offer some meager guidance on a website.)

There are actually no federal guidelines or laws in the United States regarding indoor air pollution as of 2025, and this is the same in many countries of the world. In some areas that are lucky, there may be local regulations (e.g., state, county, or city) to protect you—but this is not guaranteed.

There's no need to push the panic button yet. Just like you can learn about how to better take care of the water in Sally's aquarium, you can learn how to better take care of air in the indoor spaces you and your loved ones spend your life in.

To start off, let's learn about specific contaminants that we need to lovingly manage in our air aquariums.

Carbon Monoxide (CO)

I start with carbon monoxide (CO) because, while not commonly present, it is lethal. What makes it an especially scary killer is that it's completely invisible, tasteless, and odorless. It is oftentimes formed when a fossil fuel is burned and there isn't enough oxygen to make CO_2 (one carbon and two oxygen atoms), only enough oxygen to make CO_1 (one carbon and one oxygen atom), or CO when simplified.[42] The carbon and oxygen atoms are bonded together with a triple bond, a stronger bond than the more common

41 United States Environmental Protection Agency, "Regulatory and Guidance Information by Topic: Air," last updated May 23, 2024, epa.gov/regulatory-information-topic/regulatory-and-guidance-information-topic-air.
42 United States Environmental Protection Agency, "Overview of Carbon Monoxide (CO) Air Quality in the United States," updated February 7, 2023, epa.gov/system/files/documents/2022-08/CO_2021.pdf.

single or double covalent bonds. This triple bond means that the carbon and oxygen molecules are such close friends they have six electrons involved in the bonding process instead of the usual two in the more typical single covalent bond . . . aw.

What makes CO lethal? The hemoglobin in your blood loooooves binding with CO, about 200–300 times more than it loves binding with the oxygen it's supposed to bind with to keep the body healthy.[43] As you breathe in CO, it insidiously continues to displace the oxygen in your bloodstream. Typical symptoms of CO exposure include difficulty breathing, headaches, nausea, altered mental state, unconsciousness, and, in the case of exposure to a high concentration of CO, death. Occasionally, you'll also see blue fingernails, a classic sign that oxygen isn't circulating in the body correctly, or a red flush to the skin and cherry red lips from high levels of carboxyhemoglobin in the blood.[44]

The main goal with CO is to never introduce it into a building— but if it gets there by accident, detect it as soon as possible and get the people and pets out until the cause is fixed.

A recent example of catastrophic CO poisonings happened in 2020 in Texas during a major winter power outage. Texas didn't have any laws at the time requiring CO detectors. A number of people brought grills into their homes or went into their running cars in closed garages to stay warm. Per *The Texas Tribune*, at least 11 deaths were reported and over 1,400 people checked into emergency rooms specifically due to CO poisoning.[45]

43 Sagar Patel et al, StatPearls, "Physiology, Oxygen Transport And Carbon Dioxide Dissociation Curve," in StatPearls (StatPearls Publishing, 2023), ncbi.nlm.nih.gov/books/NBK539815/.
44 Rod Broadhard, "Symptoms of Carbon Monoxide Poisoning," VerywellHealth, November 30, 2024, verywellhealth.com/carbon-monoxide-poisoning-symptoms-4161052.
45 Perla Trevizo et al, "Texas enabled the worst carbon monoxide poisoning catastrophe in recent U.S. history," The Texas Tribune, August 17, 2024, texastribune.org/2021/04/29/texas-carbon-monoxide-poisoning/.

Other potential causes of CO exposure in buildings include issues with gas-powered equipment in or near your building, like certain types of generators, laundry dryers, water heaters, furnaces, boilers, fireplaces, stoves, ovens, and lawn equipment. Wood-burning stoves are also potential causes of CO exposure in buildings. Accidental exposure can also be caused by contaminated air leaking into your building from a nearby source of CO, like a group of idling vehicles right outside a window.

Natural Gas

Most folks don't think of natural gas as an air pollutant. However, since it is used in many buildings and homes for heating and cooking, and leaks are possible (and unfortunately relatively common), it has made our air contaminants watch list.

Natural gas is composed mostly of methane, along with other chemicals, some of which are especially harmful to humans and pets, like benzene and toluene. It is very rare to see an installed natural gas detector, so it's good to make sure you know what it smells like! Interestingly, the gas by itself doesn't smell at all. The "natural gas smell" is due to a chemical called mercaptan that gas companies mix into the natural gas so that it is easier to detect.

Sometimes, a faint smell indicates a pilot light is out on your stove, which you can relight before opening a window to air things out. However, if it's a strong smell—take serious action.

Natural gas leaks in buildings should be handled a lot like how you handle fire emergencies, including calling emergency services (e.g., 911), or better yet, your local natural gas-leak emergency number. When there's a gas leak, not only is there likely a significant problem with your air quality, there's risk of gas exploding!

When there is a leak, avoid taking any actions that could cause a spark, such as striking matches, using stove pilot lights, flipping electrical switches on or off (including light switches), and any actions that could generate static electricity. (At my house, sometimes we wear our inside slippers, drag our feet around on the floor to build up static charge, and run around zapping each other for fun. We would not do this in a gas-leak situation.) Static electricity can be reduced by increasing humidity in the space, wearing leather or cotton footwear (these materials don't build up static charge), and by carrying a piece of metal like a coin or safety pin in your pocket that you can touch to transfer pesky extra electrons to.[46]

In regards to health, natural gas leaks start replacing oxygen in the air. Lower levels of breathable oxygen can eventually cause health problems like dizziness, headaches, nausea, and even asphyxiation if the leak is really serious in a space that does not have a good source of fresh air.[47]

For a period of my life, I lived in a very old prewar apartment in Brooklyn, New York with a highly questionable landlord. One day, I was walking down the stairs past the front door of a vacant apartment and caught a strong whiff of natural gas from under the doorway. I made some calls and found out later that someone had turned the gas stove on (without lighting it), left the building, and the apartment had been slowly filling with natural gas. I was very thankful I made calls before anyone got hurt!

46 Ada McVean, "How can I stop getting static shocks?", McGill Office for Science and Society, February 20, 2020, mcgill.ca/oss/article/environment-general-science/how-can-i-stop-getting-static-shocks.
47 BiologyInsights, "Natural Gas: Health and Safety Impacts on Humans," October 7, 2024, biologyinsights.com/natural-gas-health-and-safety-impacts-on-humans/.

Radon

Radon is the 86th element listed in the periodic table of elements. It lives in the "noble gases" column on the far right, below xenon and above oganesson. The ground in many areas of the planet naturally gives off a regular amount of radon. When we're outside, it slips away into the air and blows off somewhere before we have a chance to breathe much of it in. However, when there's a building right on top of soil that is giving off radon, that radon can get trapped in the basement or ground-floor rooms and build up over time.

Radon is radioactive and one of the highest causes of lung cancer in humanity. Hanging out in a basement full of radon on a regular basis is a *dangerous* thing to do. Probably more dangerous than swimming with sharks since most sharks are relatively peaceful creatures around humans and certainly don't target your lungs with cancer. Just like carbon monoxide, you can't see it, you can't taste it, and you can't smell it, so it's hard to know it is even there!

Radon is measured in a unit called pCi/L, which stands for picocuries per liter of air. The "pico" prefix stands for 10^{-12} (i.e., very small), and "curie" is said to be named in honor of Pierre Curie and Marie Curie who studied radiation (and who both suffered from radiation sickness). Interesting fact: A common test to see if someone has radium poisoning is to test their breath for radon.[48]

You can look online to see if your local government has a radon map, which will tell you the typical radon levels in your area. Below is an example map of the United States based on EPA data:

---

[48] U.S. Centers for Disease Control and Prevention Agency for Toxic Substances and Disease Registry, "Public Health Statement for Radium," last reviewed March 26, 2014, cdc.gov/TSP/PHS/PHS.aspx?phsid=789&toxid=154.

Indoor Radon Levels and Zones per U.S. County

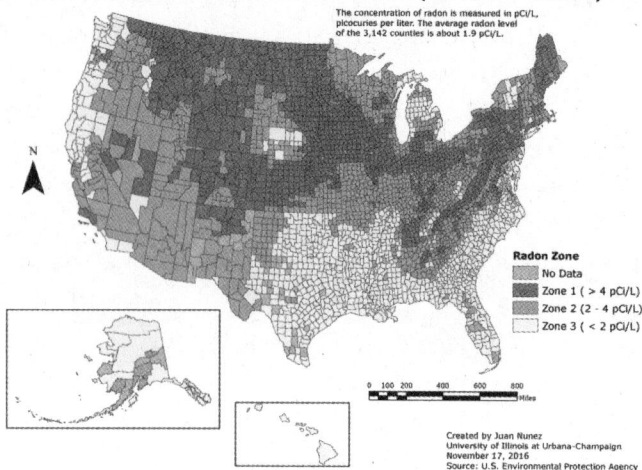

The concentration of radon is measured in pCi/L, picocuries per liter. The average radon level of the 3,142 counties is about 1.9 pCi/L.

Radon Zone
- No Data
- Zone 1 (> 4 pCi/L)
- Zone 2 (2 - 4 pCi/L)
- Zone 3 (< 2 pCi/L)

0   100 200   400   600   800
Miles

Created by Juan Nunez
University of Illinois at Urbana-Champaign
November 17, 2016
Source: U.S. Environmental Protection Agency

Juan Nunez, "Indoor Radon Levels and Zones per U.S. County," November 17, 2016, commons.wikimedia.org/wiki/ File:Indoor_Radon_Levels_and_Zones_per_U.S._County.gif.

You can see that radon varies from region to region. While some locations like Montana and Iowa are in high-radon areas (designated by dark grey in the graphic above), parts of the world like Hawaii and Australia are in low-radon areas. Just because a building is in a low-radon area doesn't mean that it is necessarily "safe" from radon, it just means it is less likely to have an issue.

Radon is actually just one of many soil gases—such as methane, pesticide vapors, VOCs (which we'll talk about shortly), biological contaminants, and sewer gases—that can enter buildings from below. We won't dwell on many of them here, but if you suspect they may be a problem in your area, you might want to get your building checked out.

VOCs (Volatile Organic Compounds)

Before I began seriously studying air quality, there was a day I thought it would be a good idea to spray-paint my tap shoes red in my living room. The volatile organic compounds (VOCs) from the spray paint concentrated in my teeny-tiny Brooklyn apartment and almost knocked me out. In hindsight, it was an incredibly dumb thing to do.

So what exactly are VOCs? VOCs are gases that are released out of solids or liquids. There's a huge variety of VOCs, ranging from some very dangerous gases like butane (used in things like camping stoves, lighters, and refrigerators) to some innocent ones like the VOCs that make coffee smell like coffee. You can think of VOCs like a big family of air chemicals with parents, siblings, aunts, uncles, grandparents, cousins, in-laws you'd rather not invite over, that one lady you call auntie even though she's not related, and a great uncle no one has heard from in a decade. Some are great, some are quite awful, and generally, you don't want too many in one place at any time except on special occasions (where you still might take a couple of days to recover from your time together). In this handbook, we're not going to spend much time talking about the nice VOCs—just the baddies.

Like radon and carbon monoxide, VOCs get trapped and can build up in rooms (our air aquariums) and need to be removed (like family members who have overstayed their welcome over the holidays and *don't do the dishes . . .*).

What's particularly interesting about VOCs is how they get into our spaces. They come in from things we bring into our buildings like paints, furniture, cleaning supplies, shower curtains, plywood, bananas, air fresheners, permanent markers, carpets, and deodorants.

What's particularly wicked about VOCs is that many of them keep being released over time. If you've ever been in a brand new car—remember how it smelled? If it was your car—remember how long that smell lasted? If you aren't leaving your Chipotle leftovers in your new car on the regular, the smell can last for months, years even. The VOCs are mostly gone when the new car stank is gone.

An especially sad example of VOCs being released over time happened in 2005, after Hurricane Katrina and Hurricane Rita, when FEMA (the Federal Emergency Management Agency) provided trailers for folks who needed post-storm housing. The trailers had high levels of formaldehyde (one of the nastiest of the VOC family) that is typically emitted slowly over long spans of time from certain types of building materials, and people started to get sick. Eventually, the CDC (Centers for Disease Control and Prevention) got involved, did some air testing, and realized that the formaldehyde levels were . . . jeopardous. They had to move folks out of the trailers—before the summer, if possible, because formaldehyde can be emitted faster in the heat. It was all a bit of an unfortunate fiasco.[49]

Why is formaldehyde still widely used in building materials instead of another less toxic alternative? Good question! Here is my understanding of the situation: Formaldehyde has been used in building materials since the 1940s, when purportedly the industry didn't yet know it was toxic.[50] In the building materials industry, it can be expensive to make changes when you later find out your chemical makes people sick. Also, some people in charge frankly

49 Mike Brunker, "CDC tests confirm FEMA trailers are toxic," NBC News, February 14, 2008, nbcnews.com/id/wbna23168160.
50 Indrayudh Mondal, Megan Groves, Erin M. Driver, Wendy Vittori, and Rolf U. Halden, "Carcinogenic formaldehyde in U.S. residential buildings: Mass inventories, human health impacts, and associated healthcare costs," Science of The Total Environment 944, 173640 (2024), doi.org/10.1016/j.scitotenv.2024.173640.

don't like change; who cares if their grandchildren are getting poisoned? These folks then find folks like Lynn Dekleva—a woman who worked for decades at a company that sold these chemicals—to make sure change doesn't happen. Lynn went on to work for the American Chemistry Council, helping them spend millions of dollars lobbying to reduce the regulations on the air-polluting (and, by the way, *carcinogenic*) formaldehyde. Then, in the first and second U.S. Trump administrations, she was brought into the U.S. government's EPA, to assist in reviewing and approving other chemicals.[51] What a world we live in.

Formaldehyde also shows up in cosmetics. In commonly used hair products, nail polishes, and nail polish removers, it can be called methylene glycol, formalin, methanal, methanediol, or formaldehyde monohydrate. Johnson & Johnson commendably became the first major consumer products company to pledge to remove formaldehyde from its product lines.[52] They pledged to be formaldehyde-free by 1978.

Wait, just kidding, it was 2015! Can you believe it took that long? That said, at least they followed through. There are still many shampoos, nail polishes, and commonly used household products made by other companies that include formaldehyde.

Another nasty source of VOCs is accidentally overheating certain kinds of nonstick cookware (such as Teflon-coated pans). When these items are heated over 570 degrees Fahrenheit, they release polymer fumes that can give people flu-like symptoms.

---

51 Hiroko Tabuchi, "She Lobbied for a Carcinogen. Now she's at the E.P.A., Approving New Chemicals," The New York Times, February 26, 2025, nytimes.com/2025/02/26/climate/epa-lynn-dekleva-formaldehyde.html.
52 Katie Thomas, "Johnson & Johnson to Remove Formaldehyde from Products," The New York Times, August 15, 2012, nytimes.com/2012/08/16/business/johnson-johnson-to-remove-formaldehyde-from-products.html.

These fumes are also known to quickly kill pet birds—so stay alert if you've got an avian buddy.[53]

Particulate Matter (PM100, PM10, PM2.5, PM0.1)

We introduced particulate matter when we talked about outdoor air. One way to think about particulate matter is as itty bitty pieces of crap floating in the air. It can be made of almost any type of matter, for example: Concrete dust is made of concrete, dog dander is made of dog, pollen is made of flower or tree matter, wildfire particulates are made of burned forest, microplastics are made up of different types of plastic, and sneeze bits are made of chunks of bacteria and mucus (maybe from sister Sally's sneezing nose).

Particulate matter is categorized by the letters PM (where *P* stands for "particulate" and *M* stands for "matter") and then a number that describes the largest size of particle included in the bunch. For example, PM100 includes a group of particles of many sizes where the largest particle is 100 micrometers, or microns, in diameter, whereas PM2.5 includes a group of particles of many sizes where the largest particle is only 2.5 microns across.

Now, how big are microns? Well, there are 1,000 microns in a millimeter. We're talking teeny-weeny bits of crap here, so small that they can stay air-bound and you can breathe them in. Let's look at typical particulate matter sizes.

PM100

These are the biggest and chonkiest particles that can actually stay suspended in air. Some are so big they are actually visible to the

---

53 Maryann Amirshahi, "Protect Yourself from Teflon Flu," National Capital Poison Center, accessed March 29, 2025, poison.org/articles/teflon-flu.

naked eye, like what you would see if someone blew a handful of powdered cayenne pepper into the air. Other examples of PM100 are big mold spores, big pollen particles, big microplastic particles, and human sneeze particles that you can see floating after a whopper of a sneeze (gesundheit Sister Sally!). They aren't usually measured or tracked by people concerned about air quality.

PM10

This is the first category of particulate matter that is measured regularly as part of outdoor and indoor air quality tracking. PM10 is sometimes referred to as "coarse dust" and includes particulates like dust mite allergens, smaller mold spores, insect allergens, dust from construction sites, dust from wildfires, microplastics, and fragments of bacteria. Research has waxed poetic about this specific size of particulate and the havoc it can wreak when it gets into lungs.

PM2.5

If you remember from our section on outdoor air, this is sometimes called "fine dust." Research has found that this type of particulate matter is even more dangerous than PM10 because it's so small it can get deep into your lungs and even into your bloodstream. Think things like smoke from fireplaces, tobacco smoke, smoke from cooking, smaller microplastics, and smoke from burning candles. A 2023 study regarding PM2.5 levels and chess players shows chess players are more likely to make mistakes in conditions of high PM2.5 levels, the severity of the mistakes increasing with the levels of PM2.5.[54]

54 Peter Dizikes, "Chess players face a tough foe: air pollution," Massachusetts Institute of Technology News, January 30, 2023, news.mit.edu/2023/chess-players-tough-foe-air-pollution-0130.

PM0.1

This category includes particulates that are even itty-bittier than PM2.5 and is commonly called "ultra-fine dust." More research is needed on this ultra-tiny dust to know the details of the havoc it is capable of wreaking, but from what we know thus far, it's likely much worse than PM2.5. It includes particulates that are the size of viruses, very small microplastics, and ultra-fine emissions from vehicle tailpipes.

Sidenote: *Technically*, airborne disease particles such as certain viruses are a type of particulate matter (generally PM2.5 or PM0.1). There are a lot more consequences from disease particles than your run-of-the-mill particulate matter like dust. Consequences of disease particles are not addressed in this handbook. There is still a lot being researched on how airborne disease travels, like: do little disease dudes cruise around on other larger particulate matter? Do tiny solo virus particles float through the air on their own? While many practices included in this handbook to address particulate matter issues may also be beneficial for times when airborne disease is prevalent, I encourage you to speak with a disease expert to get the most current guidance on how best to contend with any airborne disease at hand.

Carbon Dioxide (CO2)

Carbon dioxide (CO2) is a gas composed of molecules made up of one carbon atom and two oxygen atoms. Our bodies produce it on the regular and breathe it out with every breath, and then plants eat it.

Is CO2 good or bad for our air aquariums? You may have heard on the news that CO2 is causing climate change, and rising CO2 levels in outdoor air are resulting in scary storms, sea level rise, starving polar bear babies, etc.

However, when we're talking about *inside* air, CO_2 plays a very different, neat and spiffy role. It is an indicator of the freshness of the air in a room!

Why is that? Well, first of all, outdoor air typically has about 350-600 parts per million (ppm) of CO_2. The unit ppm represents a concentration of a substance (like CO_2) in a mixture (like air). As an example of ppm, imagine you go to an indoor play place with a rather large ball pit that includes one million multi-colored balls. Your kid sister Sally throws in her two Tamagotchis. This ball pit is now 2 ppm Tamagotchis.

Indoors, people and their pets are exhaling CO_2 constantly. If a building is really good at freshening up air, the CO_2 level inside will be almost the same as the level of CO_2 outside, despite all the extra CO_2 from all the exhaling. However, if a building is *not* good at freshening up the air, the CO_2 level will be much higher inside than the level outside, because all the CO_2 folks are exhaling isn't getting pushed out of the building. When air is trapped inside, this usually means that air pollutants are getting trapped too! So, measuring the indoor levels of CO_2 gives us a relatively simple way to keep track of overall indoor air quality.

CO_2 inside buildings (independent of other air pollutants) is only dangerous to people in very, very large concentrations. OSHA (the Occupational Safety and Health Administration) says CO_2 won't knock you out or kill you[55] until it hits levels of 100,000 ppm, which is over 1,000 times more than outside levels! OSHA says that people may start to get a little sloppy (tired, headachy,

---

55 Stephen Mallinger, "Hazard Information Bulletin: Potential Carbon Dioxide (CO_2) Asphyxiation Hazard When Filling Stationary Low Pressure CO_2 Supply Systems, Occupational Safety and Health Administration, June 5, 1996, osha.gov/publications/hib19960605.

faint) when they spend time in air with levels above 5,000 ppm.[56] However, recent research says people can actually start to get a bit sloppy when they spend time in spaces with CO_2 levels as low as 1,000 ppm.[57]

Humidity

Wait, why is humidity on this list? Isn't it just water in the air?

It turns out that the amount of water in the air inside can affect air quality in a space. We don't want too much water or too little water—we want just the right amount, ideally 30%–50%.

In certain circumstances it is okay if a specific room has a higher humidity level than 50%, for example, if you're at a fancy-ass spa with a steam room. Any classy spa will have designed this room specifically to handle high levels of humidity coming in contact with the walls, floors and the ceiling (i.e., there's no shag carpet).

Now, if a space *isn't* built to handle high levels of humidity, the water vapor in the air can start to get into things that aren't designed to handle it gracefully, like carpet, walls, your book collection, etc. If these things stay moist for a period of time, this can lead to mold, mildew, rot, and even "bye-bye book collection" situations. In addition to this gnarliness, bacteria, viruses, mold spores and dust mites thrive in high-humidity situations.

Is super-duper dry air the answer? No—air that is *too* dry is not good either! Viruses survive longer in low humidity. At the same time, living things start to dry out in low humidity—dry skin, dry eyes, dry nasal passages, etc. When us living creatures get very dry, we are more susceptible to viruses and at the same time are

56 Wisconsin Department of Health Services, "Carbon Dioxide," last revised January 8, 2025, dhs.wisconsin.gov/chemical/carbondioxide.htm.
57 Tyler A. Jacobson et al, "Direct human health risks of increased atmospheric carbon dioxide," *Nature Sustainability* 2 (2019): 691–701, doi.org/10.1038/s41893-019-0323-1.

more likely to experience agitation due to air pollution. When does everyone get sick? They get sick in the cold, dry winter months. Think: flu season, rampant colds, COVID spikes, etc.

In addition to this, and unrelated to air pollution, static electricity shocks are more prevalent when humidity is very low. Air moisture content helps keep static electricity grounded and when there's less of it, static electric charge can build up and . . . ZAP! Gotcha.

Humidifiers and dehumidifiers can be used to get humidity levels into that sweet spot (30–50%). If you're going to use them, you *must* take good care of them and clean them regularly. There's nothing worse than a moldy humidifier spreading mold spores to you and your loved ones on the regular.

Now that we've learned about contaminants in our air aquariums, let's take a look at how we get fresh air into our air aquariums to clear out the nasties and bring in oxygen. Folks who generally shy away from phrases like "mechanical ventilation"—stick with me here. We're going to learn some key Air Self-Care steps for properly taking care of our air aquariums in the next chapter. (In case you haven't gotten this yet, Sally's fish are us, dude.)

Air Fun Fact
The average person breathes over 2,000 gallons[58] (7,500 liters) of air PER DAY! That's enough to fill 5 hot tubs, a heavy duty cargo van, or 4,000 half-gallon empty pickle jars!

---

58 American Lung Association, "How Your Lungs Get the Job Done," *Each Breath*, July 19, 2017, lung.org/blog/how-your-lungs-work.

IV. VENTILATION 101: BUILDINGS BREATHE

Buildings are a lot like people. Here's a table with some fun comparisons:

Activity	People	Building
Birth/Death	People have lifespans. They're born, do the child thing, adolescence, adulthood, etc. until they're done!	Buildings have life spans just like people! They're imagined, designed, built, remodeled, and eventually demolished.
Eating	People eat foods like salads, sammiches, soups, fruits, pancakes, pickles, and chocolate cakes.	Buildings eat fuels like electricity, oil, coal, biomass (e.g., wood) and natural gas.
Drinking	People drink things like water, whiskey, milkshakes, orange juice, bubble tea and coffee.	Buildings drink things like municipal city water, well water and harvested rainwater.

Activity	People	Building
Staying healthy	People stay in shape through regular exercise (e.g., breaking a sweat 3 times a week) and doctor visits (e.g., annual check-ups).	Buildings stay in shape through regular maintenance (e.g., a fresh coat of paint every 7-10 years) and inspections (e.g., the annual elevator safety inspection).
Getting rid of toxins	People get rid of toxins by doing things like pooping, peeing, tooting, sweating, hurling and burping.	Buildings get rid of toxins through garbage disposal, recycling disposal, composting and municipal wastewater infrastructure.
Breathing	People breathe air in, then breathe air out.	Buildings breathe air in, then breathe air out.

When buildings breathe, it's called *ventilation*.

If you take away one vocabulary word from this book, I encourage you to take away **VENTILATION**.

I've even written you a haiku to help you remember.

Ventilation, by Melissa
Freshest air comes in,
Then dirty air is dispelled,
That is good breathing.

Some buildings "breathe" really well. They were "born" with "strong healthy lungs" and they "get lots of exercise." (Translation: they were designed and constructed well, with excellent, robust ventilation systems and they are maintained regularly and responsibly.)

On the other end of the spectrum, some buildings "breathe" very poorly. They were "born" with "weak lungs" and "get no exercise." (Translation: they were designed and/or constructed poorly with little to no thought regarding adequate ventilation and they are not maintained.)

Most buildings are somewhere in between—like most of us!

So how does air get into a building? How does it get out? Here are some examples:

System	Directs Air In	Directs Air Out	Allows Air to Pass In and Out Willy Nilly
Machine-powered system that pumps air inside	X		
Machine-powered system that pumps air outside		X	
Exhaust fans that pull air from a certain room and push it outside*		X	
Open windows**			X

System	Directs Air In	Directs Air Out	Allows Air to Pass In and Out Willy Nilly
Open window with window fan facing into the building	X		
Open window with window fan facing out of the building		X	
Leaks and cracks***			X
Chimneys and other intentional openings to the outside			X

*These are commonly used in bathrooms and include the types of range hoods in kitchens that direct air outside of the building.

**It is possible to use windows as part of an excellently designed natural ventilation system, which is a system that provides adequate levels of ventilation throughout an entire building without the usage of any powered equipment like fans. This is NOT the same as simply slapping a few windows on the side of a building. It involves some pretty spectacular knowledge of science and an experienced designer to get right!

***Some examples are: leaks around the laundry vent, in an old roof, and under the front door.

As you can probably tell, some of these systems allow more control regarding ventilation than others. Some (like leaks and cracks) leave the ventilation totally up to the whim of factors like the weather.

🎈

As an aside, in the world of green buildings (also called the sustainable real-estate industry), keeping buildings really well sealed is of utmost importance to saving energy. It takes a lot of energy to keep buildings warm in the winter and cool in the summer, and if you let all of the air that you've spent so much energy treating just eke out of your building, this is a huge waste of energy.

Now, if a building has been built with the "weak lungs" that we talked about above and doesn't have the ability to bring in fresh air and get rid of old air, sealing it up to save energy could result in the building "not breathing" at all. When a building doesn't breathe, the people and their pets inside can't breathe either! When making energy-saving moves for any building, you must ensure that the building also has a well-designed ventilation system. While saving the planet (and money on energy costs) is awesome, it should not come at the cost of suffocating folks. If you'd like to learn more about how to significantly reduce energy usage while maintaining great ventilation in a building, consider checking out the Passive House building certification program[59] and their resources.

🎈

Now that we've covered the basics of ventilation—a cornerstone of excellent Air Self-Care—I think we're ready to take things to the next level. I've baked the Ventilation 102 level technical lingo into a delectable story for palatability. Enjoy!

---

59 Phius, "What is Passive Building?", accessed March 29, 2025, phius.org/passive-building/what-passive-building.

Air Fun Fact:
Pop Rocks candy is basically sugar-coated pressurized bubbles of carbon dioxide. When you add water and melt the sugar, the pressured air bubbles are released and make a sweet popping noise and tickly mouth sensation while your tongue enjoys the yummy sweetness of the sugar.[60] Air-powered yum!

60 HowStuffWorks, "How does Pop Rocks candy work?", March 7, 2024, science. howstuffworks.com/innovation/science-questions/question114.htm.

V. VENTILATION 102: KIPKIP, LEILA, AND BABY MCGEE

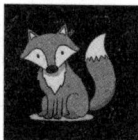

Meet KipKip.[61]

KipKip needs a new home.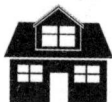

KipKip finds an abandoned refrigerator. It's great because it's perfectly sealed against rain, snow, heat, and cold and rats who like to steal food. Hooray!

KipKip moves in.

Uh oh. KipKip forgot to check if there was ventilation in the new house. Refrigerators are perfectly sealed and have ZERO air coming in or going out.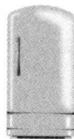

---

61 Designed by Freepick, subsequent alterations in eyewear, etc., are my own.

No more KipKip.

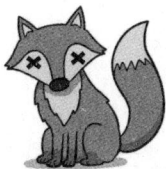

You should never, never, ever, ever walk into a sealed room with zero ventilation. It's a literal death trap unless you bring an oxygen tank or another source of breathing air. In regards to refrigerators specifically, in 1956 the United States passed The Refrigerator Safety Act targeted at reducing the number of deaths of children from suffocation in refrigerators by mandating that refrigerator doors be openable from both the outside AND the inside.

Guess what? KipKip is back and smarter now.

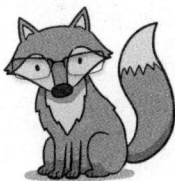

This time, KipKip adds windows before moving into the new refrigerator house. The windows will let fresh air in and still keep the pesky rats who like to steal food out! Now KipKip can breathe when the refrigerator door is closed, and enjoys the new house all summer and fall. How lovely!

However, KipKip lives in the far north. One night in the winter the temperature drops to well below freezing. With the windows open for fresh air, poor KipKip freezes to death.

Oh dear, no more KipKip . . . *again!*

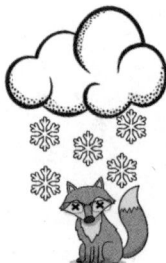

This second failed house is not conditioned, which means that there is no equipment to heat the house when the miserably cold air comes in. Buildings in parts of the world where the temperature in certain seasons can be extreme need to provide conditioning of the air used for ventilation. This means heating when it's cold outside and air conditioning (cooling) when it's hot outside!

KipKip is back for a third try, and hopefully even smarter now.[62]

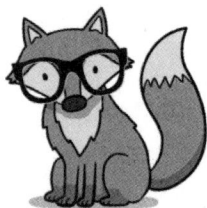

This time, KipKip adds an old kerosene heater to the refrigerator house with windows before moving in. This will keep the house hot when it's cold outside. KipKip adds a kerosene oven too, for baking fun.

The first night is glorious! KipKip makes pancakes and yummy vegetable lasagna and sleeps comfortably.

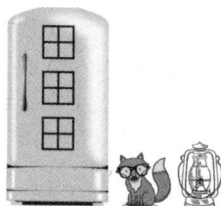

---

62 Glasses and fox designed separately by Freepick, combined here by the author for the purposes of illustration.

But, oh dear—burning kerosene for a couple of days in the old heater results in high levels of carbon monoxide, the invisible killer. KipKip is poisoned by carbon monoxide the next night. Poor, poor KipKip.

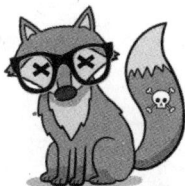

The World Health Organization has published that each year, close to 3.2 million people die prematurely from illness attributable to household air pollution caused by inefficient cooking practices using polluting stoves, paired with solid fuels and kerosene. There are many other cooking and heating options with lower risks of carbon monoxide exposure than a kerosene stove. Any time that a fuel is burned inside a building for cooking or heating, there is a risk of carbon monoxide and other baddies being released into the air.

OK, friends, KipKip has returned and has decided once and for all that it is *time to stop making bad ventilation choices.*

KipKip has recently come into a lot of money through a trampoline business and calls Leila, a cute engineering student friend to help get things right this time!

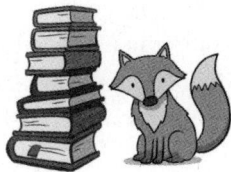

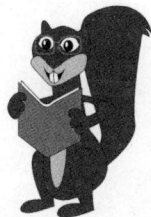

"KipKip!" Leila says. "The first thing we're going to do is build you a pipe to take the dirty air out of your house."

Leila cuts a hole in the side of KipKip's refrigerator house and sticks a pipe in it with a fan to blow dirty air out of the house. When the windows are open, this seemed to work OK, but with the windows closed, the perfectly sealed refrigerator house has no source of fresh air!

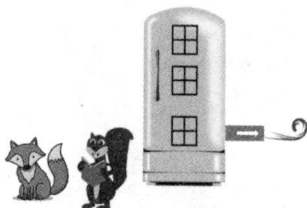

In many homes and buildings, the only way that air is moved out is by exhaust fans in bathrooms. In places like this, the remainder of spaces usually have windows that can be opened for fresh air. This design generally works even when all the windows are closed because, as you remember, air also gets into buildings through "leaks and cracks" in the walls and windows.

Leila knows it's time to try again! She decides to instead install a pipe with a fan pushing fresh air *into* the refrigerator house. But as before, this works while the windows are open because the new air coming in pushes old air out the windows. When the windows are closed, though, there isn't enough space inside for all the new air *and* the old air, so the fan gives up and breaks.

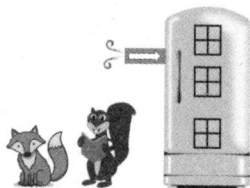

Then, a stroke of genius hits KipKip, who suggests, "Why don't we push clean air in *and* push the dirty air out at the same time?"

"Oh, KipKip—that is a great idea!" Leila squeals as she looks at KipKip with admiration.

After some trial and error, Leila is finally able to get the air coming in and air going out, traveling at the same speed. The only problem is that the air blasts through so fast that KipKip's hair looks like it got some 1980's hairspray treatment.

"Leeeeeiiii-laaaaaa!" KipKip yells over the sound of air whipping through the house.

Leila makes some adjustments so that the speed of the air does not ruffle the hair on KipKip's orange noggin, but is still fast enough to keep the refrigerator house's air nice and fresh.

KipKip's house now has a mechanical ventilation system. Leila has just conducted a standard mechanical ventilation system set-up process called testing and balancing. This process includes making sure that air coming in and air going out are balanced and that all spaces within a building are getting the correct amount of fresh air.

Leila has also determined the correct number of times per hour that all the old air in the house will be completely replaced with fresh air. This is called air changes per hour (ACH), and is a commonly used term in ventilation design.

For example, the CDC recommends an ACH of 5 in indoor spaces to prevent the spread of viral particles. This means that air in indoor spaces will be completely replaced with fresh outdoor air 5 times per hour, which equates to once every 12 minutes. This strategy aims to significantly reduce the amount of time any viruses can be suspended in the air and potentially breathed in before being pumped out of a building.[63]

KipKip and Leila go inside to bake a chocolate cake in KipKip's new electric oven to celebrate. Nobody gets poisoned from baking inside! Huzzah!

While they eat the delicious cake, they talk about things like travel, pets, and how KipKip doesn't want to freeze to death anymore in the winter. Powered by sugar and a newfound zeal for healthy building design, Leila proceeds to add a small electric heater to the pipe that brings fresh air into the house!

KipKip's house now has a mechanical ventilation system with heating (a form of conditioning). In the future, Leila could also add cooling (also called "air conditioning") to this system to cool things down inside the house in the hot summer months.

Leila was starting to think that KipKip was pretty cute. Leila says, "KipKip, I want you to be safe so I'm going to add a couple extra doodads to your ventilation system." She then adds a special air filter to the pipe that brings air into the house to make sure that KipKip's air is nice and clean.

---

63 United States Environmental Protection Agency, "Preventing the Spread of Respiratory Viruses in Public Indoor Spaces", December 5, 2024, epa.gov/indoor-air-quality-iaq/preventing-spread-respiratory-viruses-public-indoor-spaces#:~:text=CDC%20 recommends%2C%20when%20possible%2C%20to,outdoor%20air%20ventilation%20al-one%3B%20or.

It's important to understand that bringing in fresh air from outside is only helpful to indoor air quality when it is cleaner than the indoor air. While this is generally the case, in certain locations in the world, this may only be the case part of the year or never. By adding a filter that is specific to the nasties in the outdoor air in your region, you can still bring clean, fresh air inside even if it's a bit polluted outside.

Leila also adds a carbon monoxide detector and a radon monitor so KipKip will be alerted to any secret silent killer gasses that make their way into the house.

The next time Leila comes over for chocolate cake, she asks, "You know your electricity comes from the especially dirty, super-polluting power plant in the next town over, right?"

"No!" KipKip cries. "I didn't know! Does that mean that while I enjoy better ventilation, I'm making the air for my friends Sooty the Seagull and Groty the Albino Groundhog in the next town over very polluted?"

"Yes," Leila confirms, "I'm sorry to say. Did you know that after a bath, Sooty and Groty are both as pure white as a fresh snow on the meadow?"

KipKip didn't know this, and so cries a silent tear.

Leila continues, "I could get you a solar power system so that your ventilation is powered by the sun and doesn't create any pollution for your friends. Would you like that?"

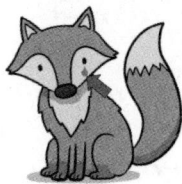

"Yes, sign me up!" exclaims KipKip. So, Leila designs a solar power system and KipKip's ventilation system no longer contributes to the air pollution that his neighbors live in.

Leila also adds a special pipe that takes some of the air that has already been heated in the winter to mix with the new air coming into the refrigerator house. This way the old air can preheat the new air! Less energy will be needed to heat the house in the winter, and the solar panels that Leila adds to the refrigerator house don't need to be so big.

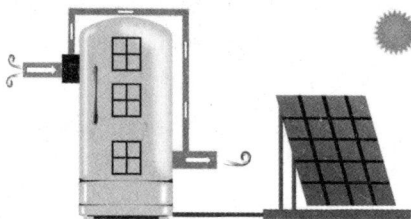

Leila saves KipKip's life many times with her good ventilation design skills. They fall in love, eat more chocolate cake, and get married. It's time to expand the refrigerator house.

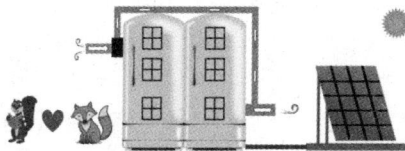

After living in their expanded refrigerator house for some time, KipKip and Leila adopt baby McGee.

Baby McGee starts to cough a lot. Over time his cough gets even worse. The doctor says, "I don't know what's causing this cough."

KipKip and Leila are worried.

"Wait!" Leila exclaims. "I haven't given our mechanical ventilation system any love and care since I finished setting it up. I will look tomorrow and see if anything needs to be fixed."

The next day, Leila dedicates all of her time to caring for the ventilation system. She:

1. Finds that there is a family of mice living in the air pollution filter, and they are clogging it up with all their precious knick-knacks. She evicts the mice and puts in a brand new filter free of debris. While doing this, she learns from the filter salesman that she really should switch the filters four times a year since they could get clogged after about three months of use.

2. Finds that one of the fans that was supposed to be blowing air is broken, so she replaces it.
3. Replaces the battery in the CO detector because it is dead.
4. Vacuums the spiders and dust out of the air pipe that is supposed to bring fresh air into the home.
5. Cleans up a section of a wall where a small water leak caused mildew, mold, and a multicolored mushroom.

Within a couple of days, baby McGee's cough starts getting better and soon it goes away altogether! KipKip and Leila put "Air Self-Care: Ventilation System Maintenance" on their calendar four times a year in order to keep their system in tip-top shape, forever.

This is a classic example of a mechanical ventilation system that has been neglected, the type of problems this neglect can cause, the type of love and care required to get a system back into proper working order, and the happy results of this care. System maintenance is vital to good indoor air quality.

KipKip and Leila live happily ever after!

Until one day, KipKip's grandma calls looking for a place to stay. She says, "KipKip, I need to live with your family until I find a new house."

There isn't enough space in the refrigerator house to fit Grandma and all her knitting needles. KipKip and Leila put baby McGee in the stroller and head out to find Grandma a new house.

First they find another refrigerator, but it is very moldy. They realize this is because it's located next to a river that floods every time it rains.

"That won't do!" said Leila. "Grandma's house will be covered in multi-colored mushrooms by her birthday!"

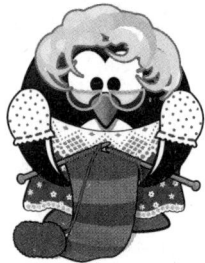

Next they find a beautiful old freezer box. It seems perfect.

But Grandma doesn't have any money to add fans and filters and windows. KipKip now knows that, without a mechanical ventilation system or windows, this premiere vintage freezer box will be a death trap, not a home.

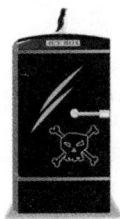

Finally, they find an abandoned electric car. It already has windows that Grandma could roll down for more fresh air when she needs it.

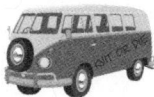

KipKip and Leila decide that they will give Grandma a small solar power system for her upcoming birthday that she can plug the car into for some working heat and AC, to play tunes on the radio, and even to power a small air purifier on days when the air quality is bad!

Grandma settles into her new home, breathes well, and visits KipKip, Leila, and baby McGee every Tuesday and all major holidays.

THE END.

Now that we've all had some fundamental ventilation education and have a better idea of how to keep the insides of our buildings full of fresh, clean, and conditioned air, what's next?

Let's talk about how to hunt down pollutants in our indoor air.

Air Fun Fact

When we think of air in our bodies, typically we just think of air in our respiratory system. However, there is also air produced by your digestive system. The average human body makes about 1 to 4 pints of gas each day,[64] which are emitted in burps and toots.

Now, where we get into problems is when air gets into the circulatory system. One of the leading causes of death for scuba divers is "arterial gas embolism (AGE).[65]" This happens when a diver holds their breath and swims towards the surface too fast. The alveoli (microscopic air sacs) in their lungs expand and rupture, allowing tiny air bubbles into their bloodstream that then travel to their brain and heart, which can result in everything things from confusion, seizures, and blacking out to death.[66] There's a great tune about it my dad used to always play on our family record player called Tiny Bubbles by the Barefoot Man from his album *Come Scuba-do with Me!* (a spoof on Leon Pober and Don Ho's homage to champagne, also called Tiny Bubbles):

"Tiny bubbles, in my veins,
Slowly moving, to my brain.
Tiny bubbles, it must be all over.
There's a feeling that I've stayed over my bottom time."

64 Johns Hopkins Medicine, "Gas in the Digestive Tract," accessed March 29, 2025, hopkinsmedicine.org/health/conditions-and-diseases/gas-in-the-digestive-tract.
65 Daniel Penrice and Jeffrey S. Cooper, "Diving Casualties," in StatPearls (StatPearls Publishing, 2025), ncbi.nlm.nih.gov/books/NBK459389/.
66 Ajit M. Alexander et al, "Arterial Gas Embolism," in StatPearls (StatPearls Publishing, 2025), ncbi.nlm.nih.gov/books/NBK546599/.

VI. INDOOR AIR QUALITY 101: SLEUTHING BAD $H!T

hen someone toots something silent but deadly in a large crowd it can be almost impossible to track down the perpetrator. Same with many indoor air quality pollutants. And yet, in the spirit of Air Self-Care, it's time to put on our Sherlock Holmes hats and find some bad dudes.

First, pause. Imagine it's a sunny, brisk day and you have nowhere to be. You've already got a cup of piping hot coffee in your hand and you're not sure what's next. You see a nerdy group gathering with clipboards, and you decide to approach to see what's happening. A sure-footed, salty detective walks to the front of the group, takes a pipe out of her mouth that blows festive bubbles instead of smoke, and says . . .

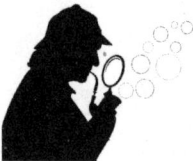

"Hey, my glorious new air sleuth team! Today is the day we start sleuthing bad $H!T in indoor air. We will all start together at a profoundly beginner level, and you can continue to "level-up" with us if you wish, or drop off at any level and re-join us on another day when you're ready to "level-up." The game is afoot!"

As she leads the group away, charging forward with a closed umbrella pointing the direction of the forward march, you make an impulsive decision to follow this eccentric whirlwind of a woman for the adventure of it. Why not?

Thus begin the lessons.

Level #00: Use Your Ears

This level is numbered double zero 'cause it's the most remarkably basic level. Do you hear an alarm sounding? Loud, bossy, blaring-wail, massive clanging fire station bells? Or a skin-crawlingly annoying chirpy-chirp alarm?

Wake up friends: you may be in danger!

Most of these alarms signal life-threatening dangers such as fire or a volcanic eruption. What we all need to also understand is that many life-threatening dangers often impact air quality significantly. In each separate alarm, there's a message you can decode related to air quality.

Here are some examples of alarms and the air related emergencies they signal.

Building a Fire Alarm

According to the U.S. National Fire Protection Society, the majority of deaths in house fires are caused by smoke inhalation, not flame-related injuries.[67] Not only does fire burn things that were not meant to be burned—like your flatscreen TV, releasing highly toxic

---

67 Elaine M. Bush, "Smoke inhalation is the most common cause of death in house fires," Michigan State University Extension, January 28, 2015, canr.msu.edu/news/smoke_inhalation_is_the_most_common_cause_of_death_in_house_fires.

VOCs into the air and very high amounts of particulate matter (PM10, PM2.5, etc.)—it is literally eating the oxygen in the room that you need to breathe. When you're escaping a fire, consider getting closer to the ground since the smoke will rise. You might also consider wetting a cloth and holding it over your mouth during your escape (if you have the time and resources handy).

Natural Disaster Sirens

If you live in an area that has a risk of natural disasters such as wildfires, volcanic eruptions, tsunamis, or tornadoes, there may be natural disaster sirens in your area. More often than not, these disasters come with moderate to significant air quality impacts, *especially* volcanic eruptions. In fact, remember how smog got its name—a mix of the terms "smoke" and "fog"? Volcanic eruptions have their own air pollution term called "vog," which is a combination of the words "volcanic" and "smog." (In case you weren't aware, "vog" is a viable Scrabble word and is worth 21 points on a triple word score.) Most importantly, though, make sure you know what your local sirens mean when they go off.

Building Gas Leak or Carbon Monoxide Alarms

If you hear a carbon monoxide alarm or a gas leak alarm, GTFO (look it up). Call the appropriate emergency folks, get living creatures to safety, etc.

If you are responsible for maintaining any of these alarms in your house or another building, please take good care of them. Sometimes they need to have batteries charged or replaced. They should all come with care instructions to help you know what to do. Also, please know that certain types of smoke detectors and carbon monoxide detectors can be set off by extra high humidity levels, so do your best to make sure room humidity levels stay in the ranges we talked about earlier.[68]

Do you know what the relevant alarms and sirens in your life sound like? If not, it may be a good day to find out through a responsible method like searching videos of alarms and sirens on the internet (not by pulling the fire alarm). Did you know that alarm sounds internationally can vary *significantly* and in certain places are not required at all? Don't assume there will be alarms when you're traveling, and especially not carbon monoxide (CO) detectors.[69]

Without blinking an eye, refilling her bubble pipe, or taking a long swig of coffee, our salty detective cruises on to the next level.

Level #0: Use Your Eyes

Of course, we've already talked about how most air pollution is invisible to the naked eye. However, if you *can* see the air and you're not 100% sure that what you're seeing is *pristine* steam (like from a fancy steam room in a 5-star hotel spa) or *pristine* fog outside (like when there's a happy cloud you're passing through in an airplane), you may be in a bad air quality situation—so get outta there. Any other type of air you can see is generally smog, vog, haze, or smoke, which means it's time to scram and get somewhere safe.

Now, how can I quickly tell what I'm looking at?

68 Maanvi Singh, "Extreme humidity can set off smoke alarms," WHYY, July 5, 2013, whyy.org/articles/extreme-humidity-can-set-off-smoke-alarms/.
69 Megan Cerullo, "What to know about carbon monoxide safety before booking an Airbnb or hotel," CBS News, November 10, 2022, cbsnews.com/news/carbon-monoxide-poisoning-safety-detector-airbnb-mexico-city/.

1. Fog is pristine white, doesn't smell, and generally will pass relatively quickly. Keep in mind, if it does stick around for a bit, it tends to collect and hold onto more air contaminants than typical, non-foggy air. As Britney Spears once said, it's "not, that, in-no-cent."

2. Smog typically has a slight greyish or brownish color to it and will *hang around*. It may smell depending on what's in it. As mentioned before, it is generally created when sunlight hits chemicals in the air. Don't underestimate smog. The Great Smog of London in 1952 killed around 4,000 people. Some say that the aftereffects resulted in up to 12,000 total deaths.[70]

3. Vog only happens when there's a volcanic eruption, so if you see a volcano erupting (or have heard there's one erupting locally), you can generally assume the presence of vog. It contains high levels of sulfur dioxide, so it may also smell of rotten eggs.

4. Haze is the reflection of sunlight off pollution in the air. This is especially common when there's a lot of particulate matter in the air. It looks just like its name . . . hazy.

5. Smoke will come in plumes directly from a burning source, like a wildfire or industrial processes. If there's a lot of it and you can't spot the source, you may be able to tell it's smoke by the gray, brown, or off-white hue.

Many times air you can see indicates not only bad air quality, but also physical dangers, such as impending volcano lava or a fire in your proximity. Keep alert!

70 Julia Martines, "Great Smog of London," Encyclopaedia Britannica, last updated March 20, 2025, britannica.com/event/Great-Smog-of-London.

Our salty detective carefully pulls a large, lacy handkerchief out of one of her trench coat's many pockets, blows her nose, pulls a hip flask from another pocket, takes a deep swig and continues:

Level #1: Use Your Nose

Your nose is a miraculous tool when it comes to sleuthing certain air pollutants. While it certainly can't detect all pollutants (especially odorless ones like radon), there are some that it is quite good at detecting. Here are some important smells to familiarize yourself with.

Smells Like Natural Gas

Noses are one of the very best tools for spotting natural gas leaks. If you aren't familiar with the smell, see if you can get a whiff sometime in a safe and controlled environment. As mentioned in the section above on natural gas, mercaptan is added to natural gas supply to make the gas malodorous (which means stinky), and specifically to smell like a rank medley of rotten eggs, garlic, and sewer gas. (Note: this is deliberately *not* a smell that you would accidentally confuse with something relatively harmless, like your mother's perfume.) If you ever catch a strong whiff of natural gas inside a building, leave the premises and call your emergency natural gas leak services (or if you don't have them, the next best emergency service line you can find). Aside from its air quality dangers, as mentioned earlier in this book, concentrated natural gas also has the risk of exploding.

Smells Like Smoke

Smoke means combustion (burning) and often a significant release of particulate matter and VOCs into the air. If you get a whiff of smoke, figure out what's causing the burning smell. Is there a serious fire? Or did sister Sally simply burn some toast? If there's any risk of harm to living creatures, take all necessary safety precautions, including notifying local authorities such as the local fire department, if necessary. If there is a less sinister cause of the smoke (perhaps you need to clean your oven), fix the cause in short order!

Smells Like Strong Chemicals

You know the smell: a pungent, acrid, stinging, burn-the-nose-hairs-right-out-of-your-nose smell. Strong chemicals can have a range of effects on the human body depending on the chemical. If you're not sure of the cause of one of these smells, *using an abundance of caution* you can follow your nose to the source and try to figure out what the chemical is (unless you're in a clearly dangerous situation like a major chemical spill, in which case do none of the above and get the H-E-double hockey sticks outta there). If you're able to figure out the chemical's name (for example, Don's Maximum Strength Bleach), head somewhere safe and well-ventilated and conduct a quick internet search to figure out if it has any bad respiratory effects and the safest way to remove it. Anytime a smell is particularly wretched and you need to clear it out ASAP, you can crank up the ventilation in the space as much as possible and add some powerful fans along with open windows to ferry that smell out of the building. And finally, as mentioned earlier, don't spray paint your tap shoes red *inside* the building. Spray paint them red *outside*. Any chemical that smells strong enough to burn the hairs right out of your nose should generally only be used outside, and if possible, not at all.

Smells Like Mold

Uh-oh. Remember the mold, mildew, and multi-colored mushrooms at KipKip's house? No bueno! Time to take precautions like throwing on an N95 mask (which we'll talk about more later) and figure out where that smell is coming from. Mold spores can get into the air and do nefarious things, like aggravate allergies and make people sick. If there isn't an obvious quick fix to the issue (like fixing a small leak and replacing icky drywall), contact a mold professional to help get things squared away.

Smells Like Cooking

Yum! This can't be bad, right? Actually, cooking is one of the highest sources of indoor air pollutants in homes, so let's take a closer look. Are all cooking smells bad for humans and their pets? No. Are some of them bad? Yes. Let's look at how to keep the bad cooking smells out of our indoor air.

1. When doing any serious cooking, always use a vent (sometimes called a range hood) that sucks air from your cooking area and blows it outside of the building. If you don't have this sophisticated a set-up in your kitchen, try an open window with a large fan in it, and turn it around so that it sucks air from your kitchen and blows it to the *outside* of your building.

2. Keep your cooking space and tools clean, especially the stove and oven. When burnt pieces of such-and-such from last month's yummy something-something end up slowly charring every time you use the stove and oven, this creates bad smoke.

3. When the smoke alarm goes off while you're cooking, this is a clue that you're generating some genuinely bad air quality for yourself. Plus, remember that air can zip around pretty fast, so the smoke particulates are zooming around and coating treasured items in every part of the house they can get to. It might be time to sign up for cooking classes (if it's mostly "mistake smoke" from burning your food), or

consider not cooking that specific food that tends to always set off the smoke alarms—or upgrade your range hood set-up to something brawny enough to suck all that smoke out!

4. Foods that don't require the use of heating appliances, like ovens, stovetops, toasters or microwaves, will generally not release cooking related pollutants. Consider incorporating more meals into your food repertoire that don't require these appliances, such as sandwiches and salads.

Smells "New"

The "new smell" usually means VOCs. Remember these guys, the volatile organic compounds (i.e., chemicals) floating in the air? "New smell" VOCs can keep spewing out of your new car, carpet, or toy for days, weeks, months and even longer. If you can't move your "new" VOC-gushing object outside until it's done off-gassing, add some extra ventilation in its vicinity to ferry the VOCs outside at a brisk pace. Some things we all need to buy that tend to be chock-a-block full of VOCs, like paints, often have a "low VOC" or "no VOC" option that you can pick instead. Another great option for certain typically VOC-gushing objects is to buy them secondhand—y'know, like maybe a used car or a used office chair—so that the previous owner has breathed in all the VOCs for you . . . poor dude!

Smells Like Toots

If you haven't already figured this out, when I refer to "toots," I mean flatulence. While breathing in toots is rarely fatal, it is unpleasant and not necessarily the best quality air to breathe.

Head Lady Detective summons a seasoned looking gentleman with a rather bushy walrus mustache from the crowd and introduces him as an eminent Flatologist,[71] here to briefly discuss the likelihood of dying from exposure to toots. He clears his throat once, twice, third time's the charm and begins:

Could you die from flatulence? Hm . . . Well let's see here. According to Dr. Billy Goldberg, toots are typically about 4% oxygen.[72] Since people can't breathe air with that little oxygen, one of the primary dangers of toots is their lack of oxygen. If a person got stuck in KipKip's first refrigerator house with *only* a supply of toots to breathe, there's a good chance they would quickly asphyxiate.

Now, there's another major contender for danger in a toot-filled refrigerator house. Toots contain highly combustible gasses like hydrogen and methane. When your air is made up of over 5.5% methane[73] or over 18% hydrogen[74] there's a combustion risk. Based on Dr. Billy Goldberg's estimation that typical toot composition includes 21% hydrogen and 7% methane, a mix of approximately 40% toot to 60% air could theoretically create explosive conditions. If someone lit a match in a half fart-filled refrigerator house, there's a distinct likelihood of . . . kablooey.

Is this a likely real-life scenario? Well, let's think it through. Let's say "a friend" gets stuck in an empty hot tub (about 720 liters in size) with the cover on. It would

71 Scientists who professionally study flatulence are called flatologists.
72 Dr. Billy Goldberg and Mark Leyner, "Passing time by passing gas, plus fun fart facts!" NBC News, March 19, 2008, nbcnews.com/health/body-odd/passing-time-passing-gas-plus-fun-fart-facts-flna1c9926322.
73 National Research Council (US) Committee on Toxicology. Washington (DC): National Academies Press (US); 1984. "Emergency and Continuous Exposure Limits for Selected Airborne Contaminants: Volume 1" ncbi.nlm.nih.gov/books/NBK208285/#:~:text=EXPLOSION%20HAZARD%20OF%20METHANE&text=Air%20containing%20less%20than%205.5,in%20air%20at%20room%20temperature.
74 Hanane Dagdougui et al, Hydrogen Infrastructure for Energy Applications: Production, Storage, Distribution and Safety (Cambridge, Massachusetts: Academic Press, 2018), pages 7–21. sciencedirect.com/topics/engineering/hydrogen-explosion

need to be filled with about 288 liters of flatulence to be combustible, and 635 liters of flatulence to cause death by direct exposure (assuming we need to get oxygen levels down to the super low level of 6% to stop your buddy's heart).[75]

Now, how does one get that many toots into a hot tub? As you learned in the Air Fun Fact for this chapter, humans toot about 1 to 4 pints a day. Let's say we're able to corral a crew of top-notch tooters who can consistently toot 4 pints a day. We would need at least 152 of them tooting all day long to make the air in that hot tub combustible, and at least 336 to kill anybody from direct exposure.

That said, it is highly unlikely to die from toots.

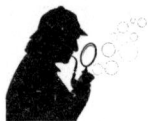

"Thanks Herb!" chortles our salty detective, pats him on the back, and jumps back into her lecture:

Bathroom areas *should* have a system in place to move air directly to the outside of the building (also called direct mechanical exhaust to the outside). Many homes have an exhaust fan on a switch by the light switch. Friends, make sure to use this switch appropriately when it's an option. Some bathrooms require opening windows to properly remove the stench and particulates associated with toots. Be wary of using restrooms with no windows or exhaust vents. These are air aquariums where stink has nowhere to go and can only build-up over time or slowly dissipate into adjacent rooms.

Many times bathrooms like these have a spray you can use to mask the toot scent. However, if you spray the chemical to mask the scent, you will then be breathing in "toot contamination" *and* an

75 U.S. Department of Labor, Occupational Safety and Health Administration, "Final Rule, #63:1152-1300, Respiratory Protection", January 8, 1998, osha.gov/laws-regs/federalregister/1998-01-08.

aerosolized chemical with questionable effects on your respiratory system. In fact, per Stanley Fineman, MD, president-elect of the American College of Allergy, Asthma & Immunology: "About 20 percent of the population and 34 percent of people with asthma report health problems from air fresheners."[76]

Keep in mind, if a toot smell is strong and it hasn't recently come from anyone's rear end, there may be a plumbing malfunction like a broken sewer pipe or a septic tank that needs to be pumped. If this is the case, it's time to call a professional.

Smells Like Cigarette, Hookah, Pipe, or Marijuana Smoke

According to the U.S. FDA, "There are more than 7,000 chemicals in cigarette smoke. More than 70 of those chemicals are linked to cancer."[77] Cigarette smoke also contains particulate matter, primarily $PM2.5$ and $PM0.1$. Hookah, pipe, and marijuana smoke is not harmless either. Remember how smoke from cooking could coat treasured objects in your house? These types of smoke can do the same! It is very difficult (and some may say *impossible*) to completely remove this coating, especially from absorbent surfaces like carpet. In the future, encourage or require that all smoking happens *outside* of your building (or for the sake of the smoker's lungs, perhaps not at all).

Smells Like Perfume, Cologne, Body Spray, or Hairspray

These fun, glam parts of our lives that are incessantly advertised to us generally have high levels of VOCs. Unfortunately, they can

76 Connecticut Department of Public Health, "Fact Sheet: Air Fresheners What You Need to Know," July 2013, portal.ct.gov/-/media/Departments-and-Agencies/DPH/dph/environmental_health/eoha/pdf/AirFreshenerFSpdf.pdf.
77 U.S. Food & Drug Administration, "Chemicals in Cigarettes: From Plant to Product to Puff," June 3, 2020, fda.gov/tobacco-products/products-ingredients-components/chemicals-cigarettes-plant-product-puff.

also sometimes interact with sunlight to produce ozone. Sure, in small doses they're purportedly possibly relatively harmless[78]—but don't be that guy or gal that walks in and stinks up a room. The chemicals in these products can trigger certain folks' allergies, so have compassion on your neighbor and stick to more subtle scents (or unscented products) when possible. As further food for thought, just a couple years ago in 2021 a bunch of major name-brand products in this category were recalled for containing benzene, a known carcinogen[79]. Yikes!

Smells Like Teen Spirit
Turn it up!

Smells Like Incense, a Yummy Air Freshener, Fancy Candles, or Smudging Sage

These products can serve as accouterments of a life well lived, and are used in countless spiritual, religious, and cultural practices worldwide—yet many of these will introduce particulate matter and VOCs into your indoor air. Warning: while thankfully lead wicks are no longer common in candles (at least in the USA),[80] certain candles release small amounts of toxins such as benzene and toluene when you burn them.[81] Warning #2: incense use has been linked in some studies to asthma and cancer.[82] So, if you use these items, for many

78 U.S. Food & Drug Administration, "Fragrances in Cosmetics," February 28, 2022, fda. gov/cosmetics/cosmetic-ingredients/fragrances-cosmetics.

79 Teddy Amenabar, "Aerosol hair products tainted by benzene may still be on store shelves," The Washington Post, November 1, 2022, washingtonpost.com/wellness/2022/11/01/benzene-aerosol-recall-dry-shampoo-sunscreen/.

80 U.S. Consumer Product Safety Commission, "CPSC Votes to Begin Rulemaking to Ban Candles With Lead Wicks Major Retailers Agree to Not Sell Lead Wick Cancles," February 14, 2001, cpsc.gov/Newsroom/News-Releases/2001/CPSC-Votes-to-Begin-Rulemaking-to-Ban-Candles-With-Lead-WicksMajor-Retailers-Agree-to-Not-Sell-Lead-Wick-Candles.

81 Zainab Nazir et al, "The unknown risks of scented candles! what science has to say: an editorial," *Annals of Medicine and Surgery* (London) 86, 1 (2023): 16-17, doi.org/10.1097/MS9.0000000000001524.

82 Lynn Knight et al, "Candles and Incense at Potential Sources of Indoor Air Pollution: Market Analysis and Literature Review," EPA/600/SR-01/001, January 2001, nepis.epa.gov/Exe/ZyPDF.cgi/P1009D5G.PDF?Dockey=P1009D5G.PDF.

reasons, make sure you do some in-depth research into what you'll be putting into your air before you put it there, and pick less toxic versions (because there definitely are some out there for you to enjoy). And then for some added luck, when using these items, flush a little extra fresh air through your space.

Smells Like Cleaning Supplies

Yes, the word "cleaning" is in the title, but don't be fooled! While a particular cleaning supply may clean surfaces like a boss, it may really foul the air at the same time. Cleaning supplies run the gamut of innocent to noxious air quality offenders. Most of them will have something called a "Safety Data Sheet" that you can find online that will give you all the deets on what is in it and any respiratory warnings. There are also product labels (such as the U.S. EPA's "Safer Choice" label) that can make it easier to shop for air-quality-friendly options.

Smells like ... ACHOO! ACHOO! ... Gesundheit!

Maybe there wasn't exactly a smell, rather something you inhaled that resulted in a strong nasal reaction like a sneeze or runny nose. You may be breathing in an allergen like pollen, pet dander or dust mites. Use your deductive skills to figure out what allergen or other irritant is in the air. If it's coming from outside, like pollen, close your windows! If it's coming from inside, like a moldy spot on the ceiling from a roof leak, clear out the source as best you can and run an air purifier to suck the irritants out of the air. If it's your pet, that's a tough situation. There are allergy shots available, as well as air purifiers that suck as much of their dander out of the air as possible. Good luck!

Smells like [FILL IN THE BLANK OF SOME OTHER STRONG SMELL]

Your smelly item most likely has some level of VOCs, and you might not want it in your air aquariums in high quantities. Some smelly items to only keep only in small quantities are: permanent markers, dry erase markers, hand sanitizer, nail polish, furniture polish, mothballs, laundry detergents, and shoe varnish. When possible, consider "fragrance-free" options or do some research to find a fragranced option that you feel good about.

To close out this section, let's talk for a hot minute about schnozz care. Obviously, if you have a cold or some other congestion-causing illness, your sense of smell goes away, so take care not to get sick. Also, remember that exercise and diets rich in zinc and B12 have been said to support a healthy schnozz. Happy smelling!

Our salty detective clears her throat, takes another swig from her flask, and says:

Nice schnozz work, sleuth team, and by jove this cranberry juice is delicious. The next level of sleuthing involves using your brain, so if that is all tuckered out from the work we've done so far today, please drop out and come join another day, when we'll be covering Level #2. For those who still have a mind like a diamond, tally-ho!

Level #2: Use Your Mind

We're not playing defense anymore folks; we're now on the offensive line. We're going to use the power of our minds and tenacious spirits to uncover the causes of BAD $H!T in our air.

Please flip to the Exercises portion of this book and check out the Level #2 Air Quality Questionnaire. It includes strategic questions that can help you find sources of BAD $H!T in your building.

Below is a summary of the questions, along with extra context to help you understand why each question is important and how to interpret the answers.

In line with our tenacious spirits, make sure to follow up on any interesting threads with additional follow-up questions of your own until you reach the end of a line of questioning and are satisfied! If you're not sure what a good follow-up question would be to an interesting find, you can always fall back on, "But wait a sec, what does this do to the air in here?"

Air Quality Sleuthing Prompts
Question #1: Is my building mechanically ventilated or naturally ventilated?
If you're not sure, please check out Appendix II: How Do I Know if My Building Has Mechanical Ventilation?

For buildings that *are* mechanically ventilated:

- Is your system due for some love and care? Remember when Leila did some ventilation system maintenance and it helped Baby McGee's cough? These systems need regular check-ups and maintenance to function correctly. Get it on the calendar! (If you're not sure how often this is required, contact the company that installed or last did maintenance on your system to find out.)

- Where is your building's outdoor air intake (where the fresh air gets sucked into the building)? Is anything funky going on at your air intake? For example, is the opening blocked by a stack of discarded, dusty toys sister Sally used to play with, or do people smoke right next to this spot? It is important that this spot remains totally unblocked and the air at this spot remains as pristine as possible.

- Does my building have a plan for when outside air coming in through the air intake happens to be polluted? You might find that:

  o There is no plan. You all just breathe polluted air inside when there is polluted air outside. As I'm sure you can glean by now, this is not an ideal plan.

  o Air that comes into the building is always filtered with top-notch filters that are maintained regularly. This is a good and potentially a great plan, especially if the filters are appropriately matched to the typical types of air pollutants in the local air and well-maintained.

  o When outdoor air AQI is Orange, Red or worse, the building stops taking in as much outside air and instead recirculates more of the inside air until that AQI is Yellow or Green again. This is like a plan to bail out a leaking canoe until you get to shore. It's a viable plan if the distance to shore is short, but not a great plan if you're stuck in the middle of the ocean and land is very far away.

If your building is instead naturally ventilated, read on:

- Do I know what the natural ventilation design requires for each room in my building so that air can be freshened up throughout the building every day? To function properly, naturally ventilated buildings usually require certain windows to remain open or at least be open for a portion of the day. The design may also require certain doors inside the building to remain open so that air can flow *through* the middle of the building to freshen up air in hallways and rooms with no windows of their own.

- Are there any spaces in my building where people or pets hang out a lot that don't have access to fresh air? For example, has cousin Dave built a photography dark room with copious amounts of chemicals in a back closet with no windows? Or has sister Sally decided to build a fort in the crawl space in the basement? In some instances, it may be necessary to relocate the things we love like a darkroom or a kid's clubhouse to a part of the building with better ventilation, like to a room with a window.

Question #2: Have the "silent killer" gas risks been addressed at my building?

- **Carbon Monoxide:** First you'll want to evaluate possible causes of CO in the building that could be actively prevented, for example an old, decrepit furnace that could potentially leak. The next step is to evaluate your CO detector set-up by first checking to see if you have CO detectors then making sure they're in good shape and maintained as described in the user manual.

- **Radon:** First, does the building already have a radon mitigation system? A radon mitigation system is simply a system that exhausts air with radon in it from the building. In buildings with mechanical ventilation, this could simply mean that they *also* have mechanical ventilation in any basement and ground floor levels. (Many buildings skip including mechanical ventilation in the basement due to the expense.) If the building is instead naturally ventilated, then this may include a pipe coming out of the basement level with a fan that pulls air out of the basement. If there is a system, you'll need to figure out if the system requires any regular love and care to keep up the good work. If there's no system in the building—has anyone ever checked out if there's a risk of radon at the building? Maybe you'll find your building has already been tested for radon and your building is "all good" without a system. Maybe you'll find no one has ever thought about radon. If this is the case, sleuth a local radon map from the internet or your local health department and see if there's a risk of radon in your area. If yes, get a test done.

- **Natural Gas:** The first thing to determine is if natural gas is actually used at the building for heating or cooking. If there is natural gas used at the building, the next step is to make sure you know who to call if you suspect a leak. The natural gas provider might have their own emergency phone line to call for leaks, or instead the best phone number might be for the local government's emergency services.

Question #3: How clean is my building?

Remember, crap in the building can quickly turn into crap in the air, just like crap on the bottom of a fish tank can turn into crap in the water if anyone stirs it up.

- **Overall dust level check**: Dust on floors, shelves, and other surfaces can easily enter the air and get breathed in. If you don't believe me, blow on a particularly dusty shelf and when you stop sneezing and coughing hear me saying, "I told you so."
- **Kitchen check**: Dirty ovens and stoves can create smoke when they're used.
- **Leaks, drips, and sitting water check**: Is there any water where it shouldn't be? Leaks, drips and sitting water are a recipe for mold (and the air pollution associated with it).

- **Trash, recycling, and compost check**: Is waste taken out of the building before it fouls up the air? Simple strategies like putting tops on garbage cans, not letting things get moldy (like that leftover food you brought home from your favorite restaurant that you forgot to eat the next day), and taking trash and recycling out on the regular can keep waste in the building from releasing air pollutants.

Question #4: What is the inside of my building cleaned with?

- **Bleach *and* Ammonia?:** First and foremost, are there any bleach-based products used or stored near any ammonia-based products, *ever*? When these compounds mix, they let off toxic gases called chloramines, which are a big *no* for the lungs. If you are required to keep them both inside your building, keep them stored in different parts of the building with labels so clear that not even the thickest of knuckleheads could ever make the mistake of mixing them together.

- **HEPA Filters?:** Do vacuum cleaners used in my building have HEPA (high efficiency particulate air) filters? Vacuums can kick a lot of particulate matter (remember PM2.5 and PM10?) into the air as they're zipping along. Certain vacuum cleaners come with HEPA filters that catch particulate matter before it's whipped up into the air, and this is the ideal situation, especially if there's anyone in your building that suffers from dust allergies. There are many run-of-the-mill vacuum options with HEPA filters— you don't need to mortgage your house to get your hands on one of these puppies.

- **Find out in an SDS/MSDS:** Do any of your cleaning products have inhalation warnings associated with them? Most products have a "sleuthable" Safety Data Sheet (SDS) or Materials Safety Data Sheet (MSDS) available online or by calling the manufacturer that will list any inhalation risks. If you find a product has serious (or really *any*) inhalation risks, consider ditching it and finding a safer alternative.

Question #5: Have any renovations been done recently in my building, or has any new furniture been recently added?

- New Building Materials: When renovations happen—like fun new furniture, new flooring, or new paint—there is a risk of polluting the indoor air. It is shocking the toxic things that are still put into certain new furniture, paints, and construction materials. If you're lucky, you live in a spot where at least some of the big hitters like asbestos, lead, PCBs (polychlorinated biphenyls), and mercury are banned. Things that can affect indoor air quality like formaldehyde (remember this dude from the sad story on the FEMA trailers?) and other bummer VOCs are not banned in most places. Just like with the cleaning products, you can find an SDS or MSDS for many new purchases and sleuth to see if there's any inhalation effects (or other toxins in the products). The following materials usually do not create air quality problems when installed in buildings: porcelain tile, untreated stone, untreated real wood, plated or anodized metals, glass, untreated cement, and exposed brick. If you're ready to take a deep dive down a rabbit hole to Alice's Wonderland in relation to building materials safety, I recommend checking out the Living Future Institute's Red List,[83] which you can currently download for free online.

---

83 International Living Future Institute, "About the Red List," accessed March 29, 2025, living-future.org/red-list/.

- **Ventilation Considerations:** When the renovations happened, was ventilation and conditioning equipment in the building protected? Construction dust can get right up into the system ducts and equipment—and it's a doozy to get it back out again! Just imagine that you were there during the whole renovation process; anything that got up your nose got up the "nose" of your building. This is *not ideal.* Your building can't sneeze to get those pollutants out again like you can, so the building systems will be due for a cleaning (or else the pollutants will be slowly spit back out into the indoor air over time).

Question #6: Can I think of anything in my neighborhood that might be polluting the local outdoor air? If yes:

- **Building Air Filters:** You'll want to find out what filters your building's mechanical ventilation system has and if they are a good match to prevent nasties in the outdoor air from coming in. Different types of filters have different abilities. You need the right filter for the right situation just as you need to find the right professional person for a specific job. An example of a *bad* match (like if you hired a pastry chef to rewire a complex home electrical system) would be if the outdoor air is full of ozone smog and you've got a filter that only filters particulate matter. In this situation, it's time to find a filter that's *actually* the right fit for the job. For more details on how to match filters to air pollutants, please turn to Chapter VIII: How Do We Fix Air Quality.

- **Air Leaks:** How do you know if your building is super leaky? Well, is there a mysterious draft in the winter that always makes sister Sally's toes cold? Or, perhaps, can you hear hissing or howling around the house when it's windy outside? This may indicate that there's outside air getting into your building. There are many low-cost solutions for sealing gaps around your building, such as strips that block air from flowing under gaps in doors and around windows. If you're obsessed with finding *all the leaks*, you can track down a local expert to conduct blower air door testing. The expert will pressurize (or depressurize) the building and see where air leaks are located using fun tools like smoke pencils, also commonly referred to as smoke pens or smoke sticks. These devices emit a steady, thin, visible stream of "smoke," made up of actual smoke (or in more air quality friendly devices, something similar to the type of fog used in fog machines). If you hold the device near a leak, the smoke will drift in the direction the air is flowing through that leak.

- **Is It Time to Batten the Hatches?:** Remember, we usually count on outdoor air being cleaner than indoor air so that our buildings can use it to flush out the indoor air nasties. If there's something funky going on outside, keeping the air inside clean can get tricky and expensive. If my building is in a spot where outdoor air is frequently bad, it might be time to seal up the building and make sure there's a rockin' mechanical ventilation system with filtration like KipKip's refrigerator house.

Question #7: What is the shoe situation?

For those of you fashionistas out there, this may initially sound exciting. However, what I'm asking you to focus on for the moment is the dirt and grime that can attach itself to the bottom of a shoe when a person walks around outside—whether it is a Jimmy Choo, a Converse, or a Croc. When this same shoe later travels through the door into a building, the dirt and grime can get all over the floors and be kicked up into the air, contributing to particulate matter in the air.

Find out if your building has one of the two optimal scenarios below that prevent this trekking in of air pollutants from happening:

1. **Entryway Shoe Cleaning:** There are mats or grates for people to clean their shoes on as they pass through the door. Make sure these aren't tiddly, tiny mats that don't actually get any dirt or grime off shoes. You want a beast of a mat that ravenously eats all the grime and particulates off. You'll need to make sure that you clean it regularly so that it can keep functioning at top capacity.

2. **No-Indoor Shoe Policy:** People take off their shoes when they enter. Perhaps there are nice, clean, cozy, inside-only slippers waiting for them to put on!

Question #8: Time to interview the folks in the building!
People can provide really great intel on how they feel in a space that can help you find sources of bad $H!T! in the air. You can start by asking:

- Does anybody think there are any rooms in the building where the air feels stale? Or perhaps there's a certain room that they don't like because they start to feel faint, lightheaded, or headachy after spending too much time in it. This room may not be ventilated well or at all and requires further investigation.

- Does anyone with asthma, allergies, or other breathing sensitivities ever complain of feeling unwell when they're in certain rooms of the building, but then feel fine when they leave the building? These friends can be considered your "canaries in the coal mine" for ventilation and air quality issues that need further investigation.

Based on what you've learned from sleuthing answers to these prompts, see what you can improve in your space! And of course, never stop asking questions.

With that, our salty detective smiles, takes a nice puff on her bubble pipe and continues:

How are we doing, sleuth team? It's time to take our sleuthing of BAD $H!T in the air to the *next level*. We're going to start actually measuring indoor air quality ourselves. If you've got the juice to keep going, load up your bubble pipe, grab a fresh coffee, and let's hit the road.

Air Fun Fact

Air can be powerful! Air and air pressure (the force air exerts when you squeeze it into small spaces) are used to power all kinds of things. The engineering science of powering things with air is called "pneumatics." Things powered by pneumatics include brakes on certain trains, jackhammers, certain amusement park rides, player pianos, paint sprayers, rock drills, pneumatic guns, and certain dental drills.

VII. INDOOR AIR QUALITY 102: WHAT ACTUALLY IS THE AIR QUALITY?

*A*s you head back to the training from a coffee stop, you hear from across the street our salty detective yell, "Watson! Top off my cran, would you?" A dapper lad swiftly appears, hands her a new flask, and then disappears into the crowd.

Once everyone is gathered, our detective clears her throat loudly, takes a swig and begins:

Hello again, air sleuth team! You've sleuthed some bad $H!T and helped the world breathe better. We're getting into some advanced levels here, meant for those who've caught the air sleuthing bug and want to expand their horizons. From here on out, we're going to be measuring what actually is going on in the air. Load up your bubble pipes and let's go—tally-ho!

Level #3: Basic Air Quality Testing

It's time to invest in your first air quality measurement tool: a basic indoor air quality monitor, available online or in certain local hardware stores. You can find devices typically ranging in price from $40–$400 USD depending on capabilities and oftentimes quality by searching for terms like "air quality monitor" or "air quality sensor."

Many of these devices look like an alarm clock, roughly the size of a kitten or small hedgehog, with a digital screen on the front and a cord that plugs into the wall. You can place them in different locations of your building and usually get pretty quick, fairly accurate readings of air quality.

It's important to understand that these types of devices are more like a "magnifying glass" for air quality than a "microscope"; you will see more than you're able to see without it, but not as much as with other more sophisticated tools. For example, some of these devices will give you readings like green (good), yellow (moderate), or red (bad) rather than exact amounts of a certain air quality pollutant.

Here's what to look for when you're searching for a device:

- In your shopping process, make sure to check that a device has a large number of positive reviews before buying. As of summer 2025, affordable air quality measurement devices vary widely in their capabilities and quality. You obviously don't want to spend money on a device that's going to give you inaccurate data.
- Look for a device that can measure *at least* VOCs and PM2.5. (Keep in mind that instead of the term VOCs, you might see the term "TVOCs", which stands for *total* volatile organic compounds and means the same thing.)

It will also be useful if your air quality monitoring device can measure:

- o CO2 (carbon dioxide). Then you can also use it for the exercises in the next section Level #4: DIY Ventilation Assessment.

- o Formaldehyde (sometimes listed as HCHO): This is one of the gnarliest of the VOCs that tends to show up in buildings. You can think of it as the crazy cousin of the VOC family that is known for racketeering, general indecency, and the reason things tend to disappear when they visit. Even though you are already measuring total VOCs (which includes formaldehyde) it's a good idea to *also* keep an eye on this guy separately from the larger VOC family.

- o Humidity: This lets you keep an eye on whether levels are in the 30-50% sweet spot.

- o PM10 (coarse dust): This larger dust sometimes has a different source than smaller PM2.5 dust.

- A high-quality sensor will be RESET accredited[84] and/ or able to meet the accuracy requirements listed in the WELL Performance Verification Guidebook section "Sensor Technical Specification Requirements."[85] (RESET stands for Regenerative Ecological Sustainable Ecosystem Technology and is a set of standards, assessment tools, and services focused on confirming performance by collecting data. They have an air quality focused building standard

84 RESET, "Indoor Air Quality Monitors," accessed March 29, 2025, reset.build/ directory/monitors/type/indoor.
85 International WELL Building Institute, "Guidebook | WELL Performance Verification Guidebook," last updated February 7, 2025, resources.wellcertified.com/ tools/performance-verification-guidebook/.

and a monitoring device accreditation specific to air quality sensors.) Of course, these higher quality sensors may be more expensive. If they're out of your budget, you can definitely still get useful data from a lower-cost sensor (that you've confirmed has many positive ratings).

- Make sure the device has a user interface that you can understand and that you actually like.
- Over time, most meters will slowly lose accuracy. Before you buy, check to see if the meter you're considering can be recalibrated (i.e., made accurate again) or if you are eventually required to discard the old meter and replace it with a new one. When comparing meters, find out how long you can expect each of the meters to be accurate before they need recalibration or replacement. Many meters should be accurate for *at least* a year or more.

Now that you have the device in hand—how best to use it? There are many experiments that you can do! Please flip to the Exercises portion of this handbook and complete the Level #3 Basic Air Quality Testing Exercise. While sleuthing at this level, keep in mind that air quality can often vary throughout the day and can also vary seasonally. Mix it up with your experimenting! One of the very best things about air sensors is that you can collect data in your space over spans of hours, days, weeks and months to spot long-term trends.

Our salty detective pauses, blows one extremely large bubble out of her pipe and says:

How does it feel to have measured air quality? Do you feel the power? We are *just* getting started.

Level #4: DIY Ventilation Assessment

Remember discussing carbon dioxide and how people and their pets breathe in fresh air and breathe out CO_2 constantly in their air aquariums? If a room has zero ventilation like KipKip's first refrigerator home, once a creature inhabits it, the CO_2 levels will go up and up and up as they breathe out air full of CO_2.

If a room has good ventilation and there's fresh air being flushed through it and old air being pushed out, then the CO_2 level in the room should be pretty close to the CO_2 level outside the building. If there's bad ventilation or no ventilation, the CO_2 levels inside will be much higher than the CO_2 levels outside. When exhaled CO_2 is not getting pushed or sucked out of the building, *neither are any air pollutants in the air.*

Enter: the handy CO_2 sensor!

If you do not yet have a device that measures CO_2, you can generally buy one for $20–$200 USD from an online or store retailer. Sensors that only measure CO_2 tend to look something like a *very* small alarm clock or old Apple iPod in a charging station, with a cord for charging.

Make sure to get one that is highly rated, where previous purchasers have left comments like, "Wow, it was actually accurate!" (As with the air quality sensors from Level #3, there is a wide variation of accuracy with these sensors, and you want to make sure you've got a good quality one.)

Before you get started completing exercises with your sensor, here are a couple facts on CO_2 and CO_2 monitors to keep in mind.

Variation Between Rooms

CO_2 levels can vary greatly from room to room. Don't assume that tests in one room will be representative of what other parts of your building are like. When you are placing CO_2 monitors, you'll want to place them vertically in what's called the "breathing zone," which includes the vertical area in the room where people usually breathe, about 3-6 ft above the floor (see graphic below). Examples of good spots to put CO_2 monitors are countertops, desks, tables, or shelves that are between three and six feet above the floor. (If you have small children, you may wish to broaden the zone to 2–6 feet above the floor.)

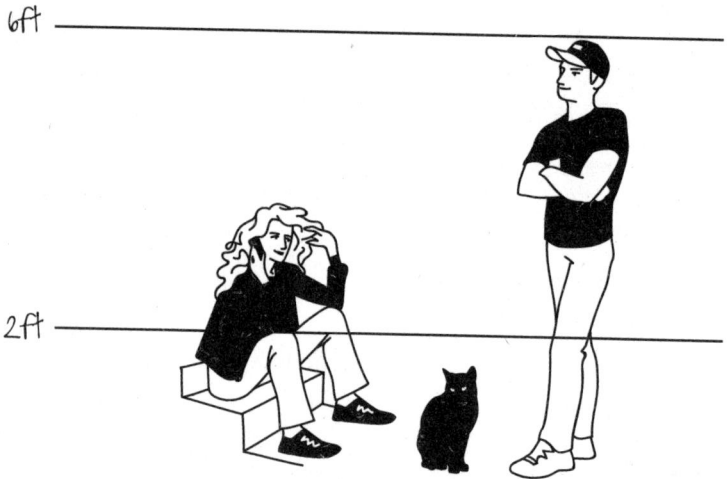

Variation Throughout the Day

CO_2 levels (and the related ventilation levels) can vary throughout the day depending on factors such as:

- Are doors open or closed?
- Are windows open or closed?

- Are rooms occupied or not occupied by people or pets?
- Is there a mechanical ventilation system on and running at a high or low capacity?

Measuring the Efficiency of Your Ventilation System

If you really want to get a feel for how fast your ventilation system can freshen up air in a room, you can measure right after there have been people in it, like in a lunch room right after lunch hour ends and people clear out.

Optimal CO_2 Levels

In terms of what is a "good" CO_2 level to compare your collected data to, you can use the table below:

Ventilation Rating Based on CO_2 Level

CO_2 Level	Ventilation Rating
Exact same as outside	Awesome
Less than 1,000 ppm	Good
1,000–1,500 ppm	OK
1,500–2,500 ppm	Not great
2,500–5,000 ppm	Bad
>5,000 ppm	Very bad, especially if a person could potentially be in this space for more than 8 hours at a time

Since CO_2 levels can vary quite a bit, when you do testing you'll need to pick a time of day for each test that you feel is representative of the time you want good quality, fresh air in the space. For example, in a baby's bedroom this might be sometime during the night when they're in the room sleeping. As another example, on the floor of an open office you might pick around 2 p.m. when employees start to get the post-lunch slow brain that you don't want compounded by exposure to poor quality air.

Now that you have your device, there are many ways to put it to good use. Please flip to the Exercises portion of this handbook and complete the Basic DIY Ventilation Assessment.

Please keep in mind that if you have made any major adjustments in order to bring in more outdoor air (such as opening more windows), any pollutants in the outdoor air could now be getting inside your building. If you have concerns about this because you are in an area that is or can be quite polluted, you can conduct some Level #3 testing again. If you can't find a balance that you're happy with, check out Chapter VIII: How Do We Fix Air Quality?

Our salty detective takes a deep breath, straightens the flaps of her hat and continues:

Very nice work, super sleuth team. This is a great time for a bathroom break and a hot drink of choice. Have you caught the air quality improvement bug and can't let go? Follow me to Level 5!

Level #5: Hire an Expert to Super-Sleuth with You

It's time to set down our air quality "magnifying glass"-level tools and call our buddy with the air quality "microscope"-level tools to help us get a clearer view on the true quality of air in our air aquariums.

To start off, who you gonna call?

An Air Quality Testing Expert!

A professional air quality testing expert should have professional-grade equipment that is able to test for a wide swath of contaminants with a high level of accuracy. They should be able to give you a flashy report at the end of the testing process to impress your friends, family, and colleagues with. If you can, get someone with a high rating online or someone that comes highly recommended by a friend.

Here are some things to keep in mind when hiring someone to conduct professional testing.

Cost
Bringing any kind of professional into your house to check things out generally comes with a cost. Make sure that you are clear on and comfortable with fees before booking *any* testing.

Final Report Readability
Make sure the professional will give you a report when the testing is complete and that it's in a format that you can understand. They might be able to get you a sample report to check out before you book testing with them!

Testing Circumstances
Keep in mind that the report will give you air quality information for a *single snapshot in time.* As you know by now, air quality varies over time and certainly from week to week, day to night, and sometimes even hour to hour. If sister Sally burns some cookies in the oven while the test is happening, the results will reflect "air quality while cookies are burning." If the test happens after the building has been empty of people and extra ventilated for a few days, you'll get results that reflect air quality "after the building has been empty and extra ventilated." The best-case scenario is to schedule your testing under the most typical, exceptionally-ordinariest circumstances.

Testing Locations

A good professional testing agent will help you decide on the optimal locations to have tested in your building. Each location tested will likely have an additional fee, so you will want to balance affordability with testing enough spots to get a useful and relatively complete picture of the air quality in your building. (Remember, by now you likely know which rooms in your building may have issues that you wish to get more testing data on.)

What to Test For

You'll need to decide what you wish to have them test for. It's truly up to you! Your previous sleuthing may help you decide what types of tests will be most useful in different spaces. Here's a list of tests for you to consider:

- **Particulate matter:** In our basic testing, we got approximate values. Now you can get very accurate readings for PM2.5 and PM10!

- **VOCs:** In our basic testing, we got approximate values for the total amount of VOCs (i.e., the *whole* VOC family). What's exciting about this type of testing is that now you can get data on specific VOCs separately from the larger group, including the real baddies like formaldehyde (HCOC), benzene, and toluene. Having specific details on which specific VOCs are high can make it much easier to track down the source. For example, if benzene levels are high, the internet will quickly fill you in that it's most likely due to paints, glues, furniture wax, detergents, or outdoor air entering into the building from near a gas station or hazardous waste disposal site (and you can take action accordingly)!

- **Radon:** If your building is at risk of radon and you haven't had this professionally assessed yet, this is the time—*especially* if you have a basement.
- **Carbon monoxide:** While hopefully by this time you have trusty carbon monoxide detectors installed, your expert can test for lower levels that wouldn't actually set off your detector but may still affect your health.
- **Natural gas:** If you have natural gas in your building, this is a great time to have a test done to see if there are any small leaks that require repair.
- **Mold:** If you have any concerns of mold in your space (perhaps your building's roof leaks sometimes) these folks should be able to test for you!
- **Ozone:** This is a pollutant that often shows up in outdoor air, especially in areas with a lot of vehicle traffic, that can then get into your space. It can also be emitted by electronic devices such as certain fruit and vegetable washers, facial steamers, and even some types of air purifiers.
- **Nitrogen dioxide (NO2):** This pollutant comes mainly from burning fossil fuels. It can enter buildings from outside (like a dirty power plant next door), vehicle emissions (like from idling vehicles in a nearby parking garage), or by burning fossil fuels inside your building.
- **Other fun options:** A sophisticated air-quality testing professional may also be able to test for things like specific allergens, bacteria/viruses, lingering cigarette smoke, chemicals that somebody has a sensitivity to, asbestos, certain odors, and even drug residue. (Ever been afraid that a tenant previously had a meth lab in the basement . . . ?)

Testing Frequency

Now, how often should you get testing done? This is also up to you! If you have a problem area in your building, you might decide to have quarterly testing done for that area. If you generally have a building-wide issue with ozone, you might want to have the entire building tested for ozone seasonally. If your building passes all tests with flying colors, you may choose to get testing done once every 3–5 years. If you come up with some kind of testing schedule—like testing once a year—remember to mix up your test locations. If you test a couple rooms every year, eventually you will have results for the entire building!

A Ventilation Specialist

If your previous sleuthing has uncovered any ventilation issues in your building that you haven't been able to solve yourself, it might be time to call in a ventilation specialist. To find them, aside from the term "ventilation specialist," you may also have luck searching for the terms "HVAC (Heating, Ventilation, AC) professional" or "building engineer."

These specialists can give your building's ventilation system a "check-up" and let you know what's going on. Maybe something needs adjusting, maybe something's broken, or maybe the system wasn't designed to handle what's going on in certain spaces these days (like maybe there's a brand new cupcake baking facility in a space that used to be a rich bloke's giant bachelor pad, and the ventilation system wasn't designed to handle all the people and all the baking). A top-notch professional should be able to get you the information you need to get your ventilation working well for how the building is currently used!

A Mold Specialist

If you've uncovered a potentially serious mold issue in your sleuthing, it's time to call in a specialist. A good specialist should be able to remediate your problem *and* help you prevent similar issues in the future.

Level #6: Install an Air Quality Testing System That Constantly Sleuths for You

Welcome to the new age, super-sleuths—it's time to "sensor up"! This is the level to go all out and have a sophisticated air quality sensor system (with an awesome interface) installed. This will let you monitor air quality across your building in real-time, 24/7.

You'll be able to do sweet things like:

- See variations in air quality across seasons, days of the week, and hours of the day.
- Get a notification quickly if there is a spike in air quality contaminants.
- Closely monitor air quality in spaces with people who have air quality sensitivities. For example, if sister Sally has severe asthma, you can closely monitor air quality contaminants that trigger her symptoms.

Unless you're a savvy DIYer with some serious mechanical and electrical chops, you're probably going to need some expert help. Whether you are building a system solo or working with a professional, you'll want to make sure you:

- Select the best sensors you can afford.
- Choose the best spots to put the sensors. Do some research on how to place sensors so that they get the most representative reading in the room. The EPA's A Guide to

Siting and Installing Air Sensors[86] and the International WELL Building Institute's "Continuous Monitoring Requirements" section of the WELL Performance Verification Guidebook[87] both contain useful guidance on locating sensors, and are available online free of charge. The user manual of any sensor you select should also contain guidance specific to the device. You'll learn smart things, like—don't put a sensor right next to a window or an air vent where nearby air of a different quality could taint your reading.

- Set up sweet notifications. For example, you may wish to be notified by an alert on your phone if there is a spike of a certain air pollutant.

- Make sure that the user interface is set up in such a way that any relatively educated person can read it and glean things like—wow, all the levels look good except the PM10 is a bit high in the kitchen right now!

- If your building is high-tech, set up a way for the sensors to talk to the high-tech building and give it useful information. For example, you could set things up so that when CO_2 is very high in a certain room, the mechanical ventilation system sends extra fresh air through that room until the CO_2 level is back to normal. The technical term for this type of smart system is "demand-controlled ventilation."

- Set up a plan for how to maintain the system. Sensors (at least in this day and age) usually need regular calibration and potentially replacement to stay accurate over time.

86 United States Environmental Protection Agency, "A Guide to Siting and Installing Air Sensors," last updated January 28, 2025, epa.gov/air-sensor-toolbox/guide-siting-and-installing-air-sensors.
87 International WELL Building Institute, "Guidebook | WELL Performance Verification Guidebook," last updated February 7, 2025, resources.wellcertified.com/tools/performance-verification-guidebook/.

There's nothing worse than thinking you're getting good data when you're not because your sensors need to be re-calibrated! Be a bit leery of companies who tell you their sensors are calibrated by a computer program. True calibration is manual—i.e., not estimated by a computer algorithm.

If you and your sensor expert are looking for more direction before you get started with this project, you might enjoy checking out the RESET Air Standard[88] for ideas. If you get really inspired, you might even consider getting your building RESET Certified.

Our salty detective suddenly stands up, stretches and continues:

Look at how far we've made it! Load up your bubble pipe and keep going super sleuth! Level 7 is aspirational and I want to make sure you've heard the opportunities it has to offer. You could become an air champion of tomorrow - the quintessential Master Air Sleuth.

She then storms right into the next lesson without giving anyone a chance to slip away.

Level #7: Become a Master Air Sleuth

The sky's the limit when it comes to understanding the quality of the air around us and how to improve it. Depending on your natural proclivities, there are many fields in which you can become an expert that come with Master Air Sleuth status! I've included some questions below to help you navigate to the start of your next air quality journey.

---

88 RESET, "RESET Air," accessed March 29, 2025, reset.build/standard/air.

Did you catch the bug for testing air in buildings?

Do you all of a sudden want to test everyone's buildings? Find a gig with a professional air testing team! They can train you on how to use their sophisticated air-testing equipment, where to sample air in a building, and how to interpret results. You can give people clarity on their spaces so that they can make their air aquariums better places to spend their lives.

Interested in building ventilation being designed right the first time?

Think of how many years buildings are around. Imagine an excellently-designed ventilation system in a building where air quality is a top priority and all the people this will impact over the years.

If you're passable at math and have the design bug, get into ventilation system design! Ventilation system designers are usually called mechanical engineers, MEP engineers, HVAC engineers, or natural ventilation system designers.

Do you prefer being in the field and working with your hands and specialized equipment?

Someone needs to install and take care of mechanical ventilation systems! Here are some hands-on professions where you can keep things running smoothly over the long haul:

- **Ventilation system installer**: This is the person that installs mechanical ventilation systems in buildings. They may also be called an HVAC installer.
- **Ventilation system technician**: This is the person that gets called when something goes wrong with a ventilation system or when the system needs a tune-up. They may also be called an HVAC technician.

- **Facilities engineer**: This is a person who's responsible for taking care of the mechanical systems (including ventilation systems) in either a single building or a set of buildings, like a university campus, over time.

Do you instead love computer stuff?

You can become an expert in airflow modeling (also called Computational Fluid Dynamics analysis, or CFD analysis) and model airflow through buildings! What does an airflow model show? It will predict how air travels through a space, including how it gets in, travels through the room, and then exits.

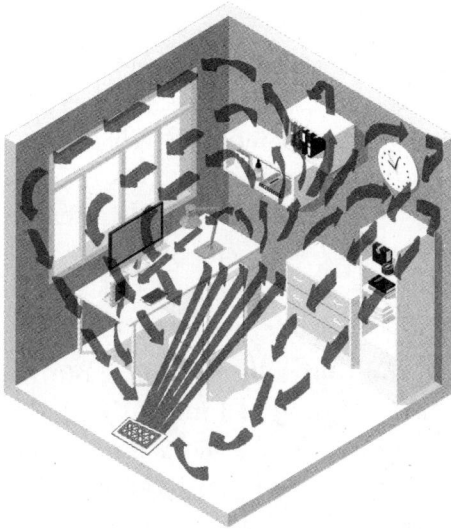

Here is an example of an airflow model, also referred to as a computational fluid dynamics (CFD) model. It can help a ventilation designer understand and compare how air will flow through a room in different modeled scenarios. The arrows indicate the direction air is anticipated to be moving at different points in the room.

It can also predict the air changes per hour (ACH), which you might remember from earlier in this handbook: the total times the air in each room is completely changed out in an hour. These types of models are very helpful when buildings are being designed because it allows the designers to model every air aquarium in a building *specifically* with good ventilation in mind. The model can show spots where stale old air might get trapped, rooms where the ACH is not meeting ventilation goals yet, and a bunch of other interesting and very useful details. Pretty cool stuff!

Are you more interested in inventing things?

The world needs new, innovative air quality-related technologies! Why not work for a cutting-edge research and development firm that works on creating:

- Better air quality sensors
- Better air filtration and purification devices
- More affordable technologies
- Large-scale outdoor air filtration technologies (that don't have adverse impacts on the local ecosystems, like wind turbines that suck in birds and spit out pâté)
- Technologies that reduce air pollution at the *source* (e.g., technologies designed for vehicle tailpipes, industrial smokestacks, and car tire pollutants)

Are you into the topics listed above, but happen to be flush with cash or good at fundraising?

Much funding is needed for the efforts listed above! Money makes things move along at a quicker pace. Just make sure to first research the efforts you're planning to help fund to make sure they're doing good work before you hand over the brass.

And finally . . .

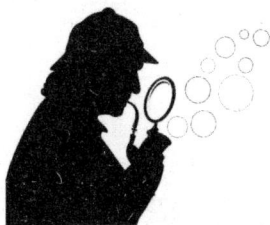

I'm back for the very last time to say I couldn't be prouder than I am at this very moment. Just remember, as Dear Sherlock always said: just like the Power Rangers, we can and should unite what we've learned from Air Sleuthing Levels #00–#7 into a MEGA-SOLUTION. Also, when you're sleuthing and you have eliminated the impossible, whatever remains, however improbable, must be the truth. If you haven't gotten to the bottom of an air quality issue yet—keep sleuthing! Never give up, never surrender!

. . . bloop, bloop . . .

And then she disappears into a flurry of bubbles never to be seen again.

Air Fun Fact

Air exerts 14.7 psi (pounds per square inch) at sea level height. This means that if you're standing on a beautiful ocean beach, each square inch of you has 14.7 pounds of air pressing down on it! If a human viewed from above takes up about one square foot of space, this is 12" x 12" = 144 square inches. If we apply 14.7 pounds per square inch to 144 square inches, that's over 2,000 pounds of air (*one ton of air*) pressing down on you—about the same weight as a large male polar bear, a great white shark, or the Liberty Bell.

Hopefully this fun fact makes you less afraid to fly; your plane is literally sailing across millions of tons of air!

VIII. HOW DO WE FIX AIR QUALITY?

*A*fter some sleuthing, you may have realized air quality in your building is bad. Aw *snap*! Can we fix it?

Maybe!

Removing contaminants from the air can be a tricky business, and certainly more difficult than getting shards of eggshell out of your cake batter.

Here is a list of the most common fixes for air quality issues and how to match them to the problem(s) at hand.

General Air Quality Fixes

These fixes are like when you get some kind of upper respiratory something-something that knocks you on your a$$ and your mom tells you to drink lots of water and get extra sleep and you scoff, "aw, mom, leave me alone!"—but in reality, it *is* probably the best cure for most things you might be ailing from.

When it comes to air quality, keep the following general fixes up your sleeve.

#1: Prevention

This is like the "reduce" portion of the Three R's of waste management: reduce, reuse, recycle. If there's no air quality problem to start with, there's no air quality problem to deal with! For certain air pollutants, it is *much* easier to prevent them than to remove them. Of course, it's not so helpful when you're already knee deep in an air quality issue, but it can certainly help prevent the next one.

#2: Early Detection

It is possible to install air sensors, such as carbon monoxide or particulate matter sensors, that alarm right when an air pollutant becomes a problem. Often this is significantly before a person might notice a gnarly air quality situation is afoot. Getting to a problem before it becomes a *big* problem can make all the difference with certain types of air pollutants! (Just like a fire alarm that *should* go off before a fire is really raging.)

#3: Flush it Out!

Indoor Air

Crank up the ventilation! Get extra clean air in and push bad air out, pronto.

- **Buildings with mechanical ventilation:** Turn up your system to flush your rooms out faster and increase the amount of outdoor air that enters the building through the outdoor air intake. (Of course, first make sure that the air you're bringing in to flush out the problem is higher quality air than what you're flushing out.)

- **Buildings with natural ventilation:** Use common sense to figure out the best way to flush as much fresh, clean air through your building as possible. You might try a big ol' window fan (or better yet, a gaggle of window fans) blowing in fresh air in tandem with open windows on the other side of the space where old air can exit the building. Or even better than open windows for an exit route, place a couple of fans *in* those windows pointed *out* of the building to expeditiously suck that old, icky air out! For this strategy to work it is essential that the air you're pulling into the space is cleaner than the air inside. (Pro tip: you might want to avoid this strategy when it's very humid outside because it could really jack up the humidity levels in your building.)

Outdoor Air

To flush nasties out of outdoor air, you will need a rainstorm or a new weather front to blow cleaner air into the area. A number of cultures have rich ceremonies and rituals aimed at attracting rainstorms[89] for purposes such as watering crops, which have the added benefit of cleaning air pollution out of the air. In modern times, scientists have begun experimentation with cloud seeding, a technique that introduces "seeds" of materials like dry ice (frozen carbon dioxide) or silver iodide into certain types of clouds to encourage them to rain.[90]

#4: Eliminate the Source

Indoor Air

Is it the new couch? Is it sister Sally's penchant for burning toast and cookies? Find the source of the nasties and get rid of it. If it's an object, get it out of the building, pronto (and better yet, contained in some way that will protect the air outside as well). If it's an ongoing situation like using a vacuum cleaner that kicks

89 Leah Flowers, "The Significance of Rain: Rain Dances & Rain Symbolism," A Public Fit Theatre Company, September 15, 2024, apublicfit.org/news/the-significance-of-rain-rain-dances-rain-symbolism.
90 Encyclopaedia Britannica, "Rainmaking," last updated June 3, 2024, britannica.com/topic/rainmaking.

a lot of dust into the air rather than containing it, or an unsafe practice such as having fires in an indoor fireplace that you've never maintained properly, it's time to update these old habits with new ones informed by your newfound Air Self-Care know-how!

Outdoor Air

Is it your local volcano? Is it a factory polluting nearby? Sometimes there's not much we can do to eliminate sources of outdoor air pollution. If you're feeling frustrated, now might be a good time to check out Appendix I: For Those Who Are Unsatisfied With the Status Quo. Here are some things you *can* do that will have an impact:

- **Transportation:** Choose a less-polluting form of transportation. For example, ever thought of walking or biking part or all of the way to your next location? How about trying public transportation? Or maybe you're able to use a car that produces fewer emissions?
- **Burning:** Don't burn a lot of stuff—and if you do, make sure that what you're burning won't release horrid toxins while burning. *Never* burn:
  - o **Plastics and styrofoams:** These can release all sorts of truly gnarly chemicals. Many plastics will release carbon monoxide and a carcinogenic poison called tetrachlorodibenzodioxin while burning.
  - o **Treated or painted woods:** Some wood is still treated with something called chromated copper arsenate (or CCA) which can release *arsenic* into the air when burned. Old wood might be painted with lead paint, which can release *lead* into the air while the wood is burning. Yikes!

- o **Yard waste with poison ivy/poison oak/poison sumac in it:** When you burn these somewhat innocent-looking yard waste items, the oils become airborne and can get right into your eyes and lungs. Mega yikes!
- **Greener Energy:** Get your building's energy from a less polluting source. Remember Sooty the Seagull and Groty the Albino Groundhog? You can install a sun-powered photovoltaic system (a system that turns sunlight into electricity), a windmill for wind power, or contact your electricity provider to see if they have a cleaner electricity option that you can opt into. Reducing your energy usage will also have a substantial impact.

Pollutant-Specific Air Quality Fixes

These types of fixes are, well, specific—like when you go to the doctor because you have had tonsillitis 100 times and they take your tonsils out to prevent future episodes.

Below are your classic bad air quality perpetrators and ways to get 'em gone!

Carbon Dioxide (CO2)

The main strategy to reduce this pollutant is the general air quality fix: "flush it out." Outside air will have lower levels of carbon dioxide to dilute indoor air with higher levels of carbon dioxide, so you want to bring in as much fresh air as you can and flush out the old air. If the CO2 levels are regularly high in a particular spot, you may need to stop and consider a serious assessment of the ventilation in your building by an expert and a possible system upgrade. Sometimes assessments will turn up simple fixes like blockages (remember the nest of mice that Leila found?) or the need for some basic maintenance. Other times they will indicate that a new mechanical system is necessary.

Remember, there's also demand-controlled ventilation (mentioned in the last chapter), where an expert can install a CO_2 sensor that tells the ventilation system to pump more fresh air through a space every time the CO_2 levels go above a certain value.

Carbon Monoxide (CO)

If you find CO in your air, the main strategy is the general fix of "eliminate the source"—and in this case, to absolutely and completely eliminate it permanently. This will probably include fixing leaks or issues with equipment in your building that use combustion (like a furnace, fireplace, or gas oven). You likely will also need to use the general fix of "flush it out" in order to remove the CO that has already been released into your building.

The general fix of "early detection" is *very* important for CO. CO detectors are commercially available and often required because of the havoc carbon monoxide has wreaked on humanity thus far. When installing a CO sensor, make sure to read the installation and care directions thoroughly. Generally you'll want at least one sensor per floor and to make sure that there's a sensor near bedrooms that can wake people up in the event that there's an issue while folks are sleeping.

Humidity

High Humidity

The solution here is dehumidification with a dehumidifier. This can be done at the building level (in a building with a centralized air system) or room-by-room with one or more dehumidifiers that plug into the wall. If the humidity issue is being caused by something within the building, like a shower room, you may need to do a better job sealing off the room that is causing the humidity. Another thing you can do is to negatively exhaust the humidity-causing room, which means setting up your systems so that there is slightly more air being sucked out of the room than air getting pushed into the room.

Low Humidity

The solution here is humidification with a humidifier. This can also be accomplished with either a building-level humidification system or by putting smaller plug-in humidifiers in each room that needs one. Humidifiers must be cleaned regularly so that they don't start spreading mold and bacteria nasties around. Talk about ew!

Mold or Mildew

If you have a serious mold or mildew problem, the general air quality fix of "eliminate the source" is crucial. Get! It! Out! The other general air quality fix of "flush it out" will help remove mold or mildew from the air, and also has the added benefit of helping to dry out any leaks that might be causing these issues. A particulate matter air purifier may also help remove mold spores and other related detritus from the air.

If you seem to be having ongoing problems and/or you have someone in your building that is especially sensitive to this air contaminant, another solution is installing ultraviolet germicidal irradiation (UVGI) since it can kill live nasties like mold spores, as well as bacteria. Certain powerful UVGI systems can even kill viruses! Zap, zap, zap! This type of system can be added into air ducts in a mechanical ventilation system, and there are plug-in air purifiers for rooms that include it. Make sure you do your research before buying a system like this to ensure the system you get is robust enough to eliminate what you would like it to. Also, safety first when you're working with ultraviolet light! It's not good for eyes or skin. Finally, remember that lamps may need regular cleaning to stay effective.

"Prevention" is also a great general fix for these issues. Any preventative step you can take to keep moisture from getting where it shouldn't be could save yourself a lot of heartache in the long run. For example, fixing roof leaks as soon as possible will prevent the opportunity for mold and mildew to appear and spread.

Natural Gas

The best way to deal with natural gas is the general fix of "prevention." If you are concerned about the possibility of natural gas leaks in your building, you can do one of two things:

1. Make sure any equipment and appliances in your building that run on natural gas such as certain stoves, ovens, furnaces, water heaters, clothes dryers, fireplaces, and grills are regularly maintained and inspected to ensure there are no leaks, or:
2. Replace natural gas-powered equipment with electric models.

If you believe that your building is at risk of a natural gas leak, like for instance it's an old building with natural gas stoves and heating, then you might consider the general fix of "early detection." While having a sharp nose is good for detecting natural gas, you can also install natural gas detectors that will alarm when this gas is detected in the air.

Now, if there is already natural gas in the air, after evaluating the seriousness of the situation (e.g., if it is necessary to evacuate, leave!), the next steps are to "eliminate the source" (e.g., turn off the source of the gas) and "flush it out" before re-entering the building.

Ozone

The main filtration option for ozone is activated carbon filters, which funnily enough are very similar to the filters used in fish aquariums to clean water. These filters can help remove some of the ozone from the air; they are not a magic bullet for removing all ozone. These filters often come in combination with the particulate matter filters that are used to remove particulate matter. The pro tips listed for particulate matter filters also apply to these filters, especially the one that dictates that you must maintain the filters over time!

The general air quality fix of "flush it out" will not work for ozone if the source of the ozone is outdoor air. In this instance, flushing outdoor air through your space constitutes a situation to be avoided, rather than a recommended strategy, since the ozone is coming in from outside. With ozone, focus on finding the source and eliminating it. If the source is outside air, it may be time to close the windows and turn down the amount of air that any mechanical ventilation system is bringing in from outside.

Particulate Matter (PM100, PM10, PM2.5, and PM0.1)

Particulate matter can be removed with a very common type of air filter or purifier. These air filters are categorized based on what sizes of particulate matter (crap in the air) they can remove. The more basic filters can only remove the "big crap" and the superior filters can remove "big crap *and* small crap."

In the United States there is a scale of ability to remove crap called MERV (minimum efficiency reporting value) that indicates what sizes of particles can be removed. For example, MERV 1 filters *only* remove the biggest chunks of suspended crap, whereas MERV 20 filters, on the other end of the spectrum, can remove big, medium, *and* teeny-weeny crap. If your building is having problems with PM10, try filters with a MERV rating of 8 or higher. If your building is having problems with PM2.5, try filters with a MERV rating of 13 or higher. If you suspect the particulates you've having problems with are even smaller (things like viruses or super-fine dust), you'll want a MERV 17 or higher-rated filter. Another common name for a MERV 17 or higher-rated filter is a HEPA filter, and you'll often find these in hospitals.

Keep in mind, higher MERV filters have very tiny holes to catch the tiniest of particulates—and not all mechanical ventilation systems are strong enough to push large quantities of air through such tiny holes. After reading this chapter, you might feel inspired to get MERV 20 filters installed everywhere! However, when you take a closer look at any mechanical ventilation equipment in your building, you might find that it can only handle MERV 8 or MERV 14 filters. Pro tip: it is common practice for buildings that have MERV 14 or higher filters to have a "pre-filter" with a lower MERV rating to catch the bigger particulates before air enters the filter with the higher MERV value. This prevents the filter with the tinier holes (higher MERV rating) from getting clogged quickly.

The image below depicts a typical series of filters used on a plug-in air purifier. First there's a screen (1) that catches large air pollutants like pet hair and dust bunnies. Then the air passes into a mesh filter (2) that removes some smaller sized particles and may include carbon filtration to remove some VOCs. Finally the air passes through the HEPA filter (3) where the tiniest particles are removed. The screen can be cleaned regularly and the mesh can be replaced relatively often to protect the HEPA filter.

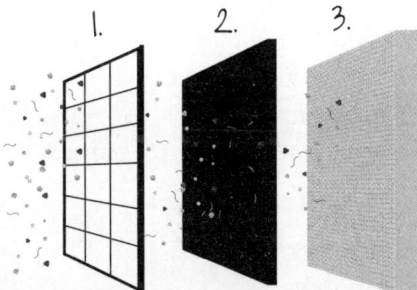

If your building has a mechanical ventilation system, filters can usually be added into the system between where air is sucked into the building at the air intake and where it is pushed into a room. Check with an expert on your mechanical system to figure out the best place for the filters.

If your building doesn't have mechanical ventilation or the system can't handle the MERV level of the filters you would like to add, you can get plug-in filters that sit on the floor. They come in different sizes for different-sized rooms. For a relatively spacious bedroom, they'll usually be about the size of a small carry-on.

Below are some pro tips on how to get the most from your particulate matter filtration system:

1. Read the directions that come with your air filter. Some filters come sealed in plastic that must be removed before they are used the first time. The directions will also tell you the best spot to put the filter.

2. Have you ever forgotten to empty out your vacuum cleaner after a bunch of uses? It probably started to get real wonky and couldn't do its job anymore because it was totally full of crap. This is the same with particulate matter filters— their whole job is also to catch crap. Once they are full of crap, they need to be emptied out (or replaced) so they can fill back up with more crap. Clean or change filters when they need it!

3. Never buy an air filter that has the term "ozone generator" in the description.[91] Remember learning about how ozone is an air pollutant and the main component of smog? There are air purifiers being sold, advertised and raved about

91 California Air Resources Board, "Hazardous Ozone-Generating Air Purifiers," accessed March 29, 2025, ww2.arb.ca.gov/our-work/programs/air-cleaners-ozone-products/hazardous-ozone-generating-air-purifiers.

that add toxins (especially ozone) into your space as part of their "air treatment" technology. A good air filtration device will never degrade the quality of your air in any way. (You might wonder, why are there devices being manufactured and sold that add ozone into the air? Well, ozone is an excellent oxidizer and great at killing molds, mildews, and bacteria and neutralizing certain types of VOCs. What makes it successful in these endeavors also makes it bad for humans and pets to breathe.)

Radon

If you find a bunch of this guy lurking around, it's time either to get a radon mitigation system installed or to expand your building's mechanical ventilation system to more robustly move air out of the lower portions of the building. Remember, a radon mitigation system is basically a mechanical ventilation system for the basement and or ground floor spaces in your building that moves that radon right out of the building. It is often used in naturally ventilated buildings.

"Prevention" is a general fix that can be employed while a building is being built. In areas that have higher levels of radon, a radon barrier can be installed. This is a giant sheet of protective membrane goodness that gets rolled out over the soil before a concrete foundation is poured to prevent gasses from seeping into the building from below.

When it comes to radon, it is also possible to employ "detection." It's fairly easy to find a radon testing kit online these days and conduct a radon test yourself! This will give you a value specific to your building (which may be different from other buildings in your area). It is generally also possible to hire someone to do a radon test for you. If your building is in an area where radon levels are especially high, you might consider commercially available radon monitors that will constantly monitor radon levels and alarm when radon levels exceed a certain threshold. These can be helpful indicators that a radon mitigation or prevention system has a problem.

VOCs (also called TVOCs)

These are unfortunately trickier to get out of the air than particulate matter. The General Air Quality Fixes section includes the best strategies for these nasties, specifically: "flush it out" and "eliminate the source."

In addition to those fixes, you can use an activated carbon filter, just like for ozone. As with ozone, it will remove some of the VOCs, but not all.

Of course, sometimes it's the case that we land in spots where we can't fix the air around us. Maybe we're in a situation we could not have predicted, like a volcano eruption on vacation, or we need to drive through a town where the shoe polish factory just caught on fire and plumes of toxic fumes are passing over. Things happen! The next chapter covers how to prepare for these situations.

Air Fun Fact

Did you know that when you lose weight, you breathe most of it out? When fat breaks down, it primarily breaks into water and carbon. The water you pee and sweat out, and the carbon you breathe out. Another reason to have healthy lungs![92]

92 Ruben Meerman and Andrew J. Brown, "When somebody loses weight, where does the fat go?" BMJ 349 (2014): g7257, doi.org/10.1136/bmj.g7257.

IX. HOW TO PREPARE FOR BAD AIR

Sometimes air is bad—for reasons known, unknown, or this, that, and the other thing that's out of our control. The bad air could be outside, inside, or both.

Here is a list of preparation steps you can take to protect yourself and your friends, family, and pets in the event that particularly bad air quality can't be avoided. These recommendations may need to be modified for people with lung sensitivities, including children, the elderly, asthmatics, and people with other lung diseases. A trusted medical expert can help with modifications.

Here we go!

Regularly Monitor the Air Situation

None of us want to be the last one in the pool to find out that a kid pooped, and we've been swimming in poopy pool water for the last 20 minutes. We want to be the *first* out of the pool. To be the first one, we need to regularly monitor the situation and have the most current data.

Some governments will send warnings publicly when air quality gets quite dire, but oftentimes by this point, everyone has already been exposed to the air pollution (perhaps even a large dose of it).

Instead, why not:

- Check the outdoor air quality *every day* when you check the weather.
- Install an app on your phone that will give you the AQI no matter what your location is. In some phone apps, you can set up sweet alerts that go off anytime air quality reaches an AQI threshold that you want to know about; for example, "100," which is the AQI value on the border between "yellow" and "orange" on the AQI spectrum.
- Reach at least Level #3: Basic Air Quality Testing as discussed in "Chapter VII: Indoor Air Quality 102" so that you have at least one basic indoor air quality measuring device on hand. Consider having at least one in any spaces that you and your loved ones spend lots of time in. Certain devices allow you to set alarms when air quality goes above thresholds in your inside spaces.

Change Location

Why swim in the poopy pool when you can head on over to the clean wave pool? Many times, the best strategy when air quality is bad is to get up and simply move to a better location.

Where is that place? Knowing where to go may require some advanced legwork!

Sometimes it's as easy as heading *inside,* like in the case where there are raging wildfires a couple cities away and tons of smoke has managed to blow into your area. As long as you stay indoors with the windows closed, you can avoid the smoke.

Sometimes it's as easy as heading *outside*, like in the case where some chump mixed bleach and ammonia together in an effort to clean a floor super well, and now toxic chemical fumes are wafting through your building.

In other situations, it may require moving a significant geographical distance either temporarily, like if an event occurs in your area like the 1952 Great Smog of London that lasted for four days and killed thousands of people, *or* permanently, like if you have asthma and your city regularly has AQI days in the "red" (and this isn't forecast to change in the next couple years).

Have PPE (Personal Protective Equipment) On Hand

There are situations where you need to immediately protect yourself from poor air quality. In these cases, we can *wear* air quality protective gear, sometimes referred to as PPE (Personal Protective Equipment).

Below are types of PPE and when to wear them. They're organized from the most common air quality circumstances to the most extreme:

"Significant" Conditions

Conditions where a moderate amount of air filtration is needed. Some examples are:

- Throwing on an **N95 mask** before walking across town to get a yummy bagel because there's currently an "air quality alert" for particulate matter (and I'm hungry).

- Sister Sally needs to get to school on the same day that the farms nearby are spraying fertilizers. Mom drives her instead of letting her bike and makes sure that the car is **filtering and recirculating air** instead of bringing any air from outside into the car.
- A construction worker is working at a site not too far from where wildfires have broken out, and smoke is wafting through the construction site. They throw on a **disposable respirator** that is available through their company to protect them from the smoke.

"Extreme" Conditions

These are conditions where it is necessary to have *major* air filtration capacity as part of your PPE. Some examples are:

- a worker traveling to clean up a dangerous chemical spill wearing a HAZMAT suit fitted with a **powered air purifying respirator (PAPR)**
- a combatant fighting in a war zone who is wearing a **gas mask** because there is an imminent risk of tear gas or another chemical agent being used
- a doctor working closely with patients in an area experiencing a major deadly disease outbreak (such as ebola) wearing a **respirator** to prevent themselves from being exposed to the disease

"Super Extreme" Conditions

These are conditions where the air is so unbreathable that it is necessary to bring good air along with you as part of your PPE. Some examples are:

- a scuba diver diving for treasure who brings a **scuba tank**
- a fireman running to save a kitten in a burning building who brings **air tanks**

- a plane experiencing a significant drop in cabin pressure and the **oxygen masks** drop so passengers can have oxygen to breathe

As I said before, most of us only need to prepare for the "significant" conditions on this scale. If you anticipate being exposed to air conditions that are more extreme in your area or wish to learn more about PPE used in more extreme scenarios, consider getting trained in an emergency response profession where they will guide you on how to correctly use more intensive types of air PPE.

See below for a couple types of relatively easy-to-access PPE that you may want to have on hand if you ever find yourself in "significant" air conditions.[93]

N95 Masks

Many of us have N95 masks on hand from the COVID-19 pandemic. Great news: they can *also* be used to protect you when particulate matter counts are very high, since they can filter about 95% of particles down to size 0.3 microns (PM0.3)! This means they will filter out PM10 and a good amount of PM2.5. Happily, this means they will also filter:

- airborne allergens (such as dust mite allergens and pet dander), which are typically 1–30 microns in size (PM1–PM30)
- pollen, which is usually about 30 microns in size (PM30)
- most mold spores, which are typically 4–20 microns in size (PM4–PM20)

---

93 U.S. Centers for Disease Control and Prevention National Personal Protective Technology Laboratory (NPPTL), "NIOSH-Approved Particulate Filtering Facepiece Respirators", last updated November 5, 2024, cdc.gov/niosh/npptl/topics/respirators/disp_part/default.html.

KN95 Masks

These are masks that are certified by a Chinese standard. They are often more affordable and, very importantly, more comfortable to wear than the N95 masks. The FDA has posted a list of KN95 masks that have tested as well as N95 masks.[94] If you don't see a particular KN95 manufacturer on this list, their mask may not perform as well as a regular N95 mask and you might look for a different brand (or just get an N95 mask).

P95 Masks

A P95 mask can do what an N95 mask can do and it can also protect you specifically from oil particulates in the air (i.e., air contaminants from oil and gas operations, industrial activities, or cooking). If you're not worried about oil particulates in the air, this mask may be overkill.

Surgical Masks

These masks are designed to filter out germs that the wearer may breathe out on other people. If you're strictly trying to protect yourself from breathing in air pollutants outside, these will help, but not as well as an N95 mask. That said, if you're trying to prevent yourself from spreading COVID-19 or a nasty cold to your family, this could be a great mask option for you!

Cloth Masks

Cloth masks have a very large range of effectiveness. They have been tested to remove <30%–91% of particulate matter from the air that's being breathed in by the wearer.[95] Cloth masks that perform

---

94 U.S. Food & Drug Administration, "Personal Protective Equipments EUAs," last updated November 12, 2024, 2023, fda.gov/medical-devices/covid-19-emergency-use-authorizations-medical-devices/personal-protective-equipment-euas#appendixa.
95 Amy V. Mueller et al, "Quantitative Method for Comparative Assessment of Particle Removal Efficiency of Fabric Masks as Alternatives to Standard Surgical Masks for PPE," *Matter* 3,3 (2020): 950-962, doi.org/10.1016/j.matt.2020.07.006.

better usually have a tighter fit, more protective layers, and a layer with very tiny holes (like a breathable coffee filter). If you can't find an N95 mask and you're in a pinch, you can make a cloth mask for some added protection. Matthew McConaughey has a video with a coffee filter bandana mask that is worth checking out if you're not sure where to start.[96] (It just takes one bandana, one coffee filter, two rubber bands and no special skills like sewing.) If you're making a homemade mask, triple-check to make sure whatever type of home filter material you grab is something you can actually breathe through, that won't get weird chemicals on your face (like certain dryer sheets), and that won't give off any kind of fiberglass particles for you to breathe in.

Masks with an Activated Carbon Filter

These will cut down the amount of VOCs and ozone in the air that you might breathe in. Keep in mind that they are not nearly as efficient as the N95 masks; in fact, many won't even remove as much as 50% of the VOCs in the air. That said, less VOCs in the lungs *are* less VOCs in the lungs, and sometimes we need the small wins!

Gas Masks

If you like to be prepared for *all possible situations*, you might delve into the world of commercially available gas masks and stock up on a couple that remove high levels of particulates and chemicals from the air. There are even some types that are designed to filter out carbon monoxide. As with all PPE, make sure you're wearing the mask correctly and there are no leaks around your nose or chin.

Gas masks are particularly handy if you're doing something like spray painting your tap shoes red, and the only place you can do it is in your tiny living room with the windows closed . . .

---

96 Good Morning America, "Matthew McConaughey teaches us how to make a face mask," GMA Digital, April 13, 2020, 59 sec., youtube.com/watch?v=I18Q_48ODBQ.

Strengthen Your Respiratory System

Sometimes it's the kid next to you that pees in the pool, and you're affected no matter how much you've prepared. In these cases, the air pollution *is* getting into your lungs.

At this point we reach a simple truth that, in general, strong lungs will perform better when flooded with air pollution than weak lungs. We all start with a different set of lungs. Some of us had childhood asthma, some of us have marathoner lungs, some of us are infants with tiny little baby lungs, some of us have been smokers, some of us come from a strong family tradition of yodeling. We start from where we start from—and even those of us with relatively healthy respiratory systems can work to make our lungs stronger!

Based on where you're starting from, different lung strengthening practices will be better for you. Please use caution and consult a medical expert if you're unsure of what will jam with your particular respiratory system.

Let's start with eliminating significant hindrances to your respiratory system:

Quit Smoking

OK, if you're a smoker (full-time, part-time, or occasional, using vapes, corn-pipes, hookah, doobies, etc.), this might not feel like a fun place to start. Just remember, smoking is a voluntary form of bringing air pollution directly into your lungs, which can seriously weaken them. According to the American Cancer Society, a smoker's risk of coronary heart disease doesn't drop to the same risk as a non-smoker until 15 years after they quit! Better news: the carbon monoxide (CO) levels in a smoker's blood should drop to normal just a couple days after quitting.[97]

Rigorously Manage Your Allergies

Allergies plus air pollution is a double whammy on the respiratory system. If there's anything you can do to minimize your current allergy situation (especially anything preventative), get into the habit of doing it on a regular basis. When your system is less reactionary, it can handle air pollution better. Your regimen might include things like:

- Get **tested for allergies** to figure out what exactly you're allergic to, if you haven't yet.
- For **seasonal allergies,** remember to start taking your seasonal allergy medication at least a couple weeks *before* the season starts so your body is ready.
- For **long-term allergies**, regularly take any prescribed allergy medication and/or commit to regular allergy shots.
- For **dust mite allergies**, get dust mite covers for your pillow and mattress, a HEPA filter vacuum, and a particulate matter air purifier for your bedroom.
- For **pollen allergies**, remember to keep windows and doors closed as much as possible during pollen season, get a particulate matter air purifier for your home, and wear N95 masks outside when the pollen is especially high.

Do Your Best to Avoid Respiratory Illnesses

Whether it's COVID-19, the flu, or a cold, no one wants to be sniffly and coughing up a lung—especially when there's a bad air quality event like a volcano erupting nearby. Follow what works for you to stave off the plagues of our time! You can try things like

---

97 American Cancer Society, "Health Benefits of Quitting Smoking Over Time," last revised October 28, 2024, cancer.org/healthy/stay-away-from-tobacco/benefits-of-quitting-smoking-over-time.html.

avoiding sick folks, eating healthy (get your vitamins and minerals!), supplementing with immune system boosting products when you feel an illness coming on, and receiving preventative vaccines (like for the flu, whooping cough, and COVID-19).

Sleuth Out Bad Habits That Impede Your Breathing

Do you hold your breath or breathe shallowly when you're stressed? Do you wear tight clothes that impede you from taking in a full breath, like a corset? Do you wear nose jewelry so gigantic it blocks a nasal passage? Try to eliminate any habits and physical obstructions that impede your natural breathing.

Eat Healthy Foods Rich with Antioxidants

Air pollution can cause too many oxidants in the body, which result in free radicals in your system that can target lung cells. Foods rich in antioxidants can help stave off the effects of these extra free radicals. There are lots of yummy high antioxidant food options like berries, sweet potatoes, dark chocolate, pumpkin seeds, walnuts, and artichoke hearts, as well as delicious drink options like coffee, red wine, green tea, and pomegranate juice. The internet is chock-a-block full of antioxidant-rich food and drink options to explore!

Now let's talk about ways to strengthen your lungs! It goes without saying, though I'll say it anyway: *please only pursue the strengthening exercises below in areas with good air quality, and consult with your doctor before beginning any new exercise regime.* Have fun!

Classic Cardiovascular Exercise

Jumping jacks! Jogging! Calisthenics! Swimming! Bicycling! The boot camp shenanigans they show in the army movies! Any exercise that gets your heart rate up will contribute to strong, healthy lungs.

Humming

Take some nice, big breaths and try continuously humming for a few minutes a day. You can hum whatever you please—perhaps a show tune, a rock opera, the latest pop hit, or even just a single note! Each time you breathe in, try to explore how big your lungs actually are in all directions (up, down, forward, back, side-to-side). Not only can this help strengthen your lungs, it can help clear out nasal passages if you let the humming vibrations in your nose really get going. Cleared out nasal passages means bigger channels to get air in and out of your lungs quickly. Also, a classic side-effect of humming is that it tends to reduce anxiety.[98] If you get bored of regular humming, try the kazoo!

Singing

Time to belt it out. You can join a choir, sing in the shower, rock at karaoke, or take a singing lesson even if you have zero talent. Per studies, singers have markedly larger lung capacity than non-singers.[99] Believe me, this has virtually no correlation with their singing talent! Major bonus points if you study with an opera singer; they are the Olympians of singers and masters of expanding breathing capacities.

Practice Relaxation in Stressful Situations

As many an asthmatic will tell you, when it starts to feel hard to breathe, it is very easy to panic. The last thing we want to do in a

---

98 Gunjan Trivedi et al, "Humming (Simple Bhramari Pranayama) as a Stress Buster: A Holter-Based Study to Analyze Heart Rate Variability (HRV) Parameters During Bhramari, Physical Activity, Emotional Stress, and Sleep," *Cureus* 15, 4 e37527 (2023), doi.org/10.7759/cureus.37527.

99 Abyan Irzaldy et al, "Lung Vital Capacity of Choir Singers and Nonsingers: A Comparative Study," *Journal of Voice: Official Journal of the Voice Foundation* 30, 6 (2016): 717-720. doi.org/10.1016/j.jvoice.2015.08.008.

situation where the air quality is dicey is to panic. In an extreme situation like a house fire, having a calm head on our shoulders and an awareness of the best way to handle our human air needs in the moment can be the difference between life or death.

Many people in this busy world of ours live with the mantra, "I'll relax when I'm dead." In terms of Air Self-Care, this is a real miss, since relaxation is a *crucial* tool to master in preparation for any situation where you're having difficulty breathing. Typical non-relaxed stress reactions to these situations can include:

Tensing Up Muscles

When you breathe in, the diaphragm must relax and your torso—including shoulders, chest muscles, and back muscles—must expand to let a certain volume of air in. If any of these elements are tense, they will literally physically limit the amount of air that is able to enter your body. To test if any of these muscles are tense, simply take in a giant breath and try to sense if any muscles are constricting.

Did you know, when you breathe out it's called "exhalation" and when you breathe in it's called "inspiration." Relaxed torso muscles literally allow for more *inspiration*!

Overbreathing (Hyperventilation)

This is a condition where a person starts breathing too much, which causes an imbalance of oxygen and CO_2 in the bloodstream (too much CO_2). This can result in dizziness, shortness of breath, tingling in the fingers, and myriad other issues that you don't want to be messing around with during a bad air quality event—or ever!

Reactionary Decision-Making

In an emergency, I'd rather be making informed decisions than reacting wildly, wouldn't you? No one wants to be a silly goose in a fire situation, running around and screaming instead of making the more informed choice to get close to the floor in order to breathe better air and find a safe escape route! Relaxation can put you in a better mind-space to make well-informed decisions in life-or-death situations.

There are many ways to learn about, study, and practice relaxation. I encourage you to explore and figure out what works best for you, since everyone is very different in this arena. Here are some ideas for restorative relaxation practices that may bring your average stress level down when you do them regularly:

- long walks
- cardiovascular workouts
- restorative yoga
- meditation
- humming or singing
- contemplative "maker" hobbies
- cognitive behavioral therapy with a qualified therapist
- contemplative food making
- "self-care" practices such as regular visits to the spa
- restorative treatments such as massage and reiki

As stated above, the following are potential strategies to consider—and as always, please consult with a qualified physician before beginning any new practices or treatments.

If you want to put your relaxation skills to the test in some relatively safe, high-stakes situations, good for you! You inspire me. Here are some realms that are great for practicing keeping a cool head and unimpeded natural breathing:

- interactive martial arts
- fast-paced competitive sports

- fast-paced competitive gaming such as board games, capture the flag, online gaming, speed chess, and that card game where you slap people's hands
- clubs where you take turns giving speeches to audiences
- improv acting

That takes us to the end of our chapter on preparation for bad air quality events. Nice work! It's time to move on to the final chapter that summarizes what we've learned.

Air Fun Fact

Phytoplankton in the ocean make over 70% of our world's oxygen! What a great reason to take excellent care of our oceans![100]

100 National Geographic, "Save the Plankton, Breathe Freely," accessed March 29, 2025, media.nationalgeographic.org/assets/activity/assets/save-the-plankton-breathe-freely-1.pdf.

X. CONCLUSION

We've made it to the end of our journey together and have learned a lot about Air Self-Care!

Now that you've read through the handbook, please recall some of the important stats mentioned throughout the book:

1. Air pollution kills significantly more people per year than peak COVID, war and conflicts, and shark attacks.
2. Indoor air can be far more polluted than outdoor air. Each room in a building needs to be considered as a separate air aquarium, with care taken to maintain oxygen levels and reduce pollution levels.
3. Air pollution affects the body in many ways, all contributing to adverse health effects, since it can go directly through the lungs into the bloodstream and impact organs including your brain.

These are all great reasons to get into action on your Air Self-Care! If this book was a bit of a wake-up call and you're really just not sure where to get started, here's a five-step plan that should jump-start your Air Self-Care journey and have you ready and prepared for the average day, for $50 or less (especially if you're a savvy shopper or already have some of the items below on hand):

1. **Check outdoor air quality regularly**. You can find it online by searching, "What is the AQI near me right now?" or by using a cool air quality app on your phone. Remember: green is good! If on any given day it isn't green (or yellow if you feel confident in your respiratory system), make plans that don't involve being outside a lot, etc.

2. **Open a window every day**. When the AQI is good (green) and it's not incredibly humid outside, open some windows! Invest in at least one window fan to push air through your space. Remember, your building needs to breathe well so that *you* can breathe well.

3. **Have N95 masks on hand.** Have these dudes on hand and wear them when the AQI isn't green and PM2.5 or PM10 is high. Other great times to wear these are:
   o When you have to go outside during pollen season
   o When it's super-duper dry and you have a respiratory sensitivity to dry air. The masks will help trap the humidity from your breath.
   o When you're sick and don't want to contribute to particulate matter in the air

4. **Don't bring air polluters inside**. Indoor air can be damn well near impossible to clean once it's polluted—so keep it clean! Don't bring toxic chemicals or dusty, dirty, or smelly stuff into the building. When the air quality is reduced, get the related air pollutants out of the building, pronto.

5. **Keep your lungs strong!** This world is unfortunately not moving very quickly towards pristine, clean air and water for all—so work on getting a "buffer" respiratory system to handle what's out there.

Once you're on a roll with these five items, re-read the handbook and keep adding to your Air Self-Care regimen until you feel like you've got a solid handle on your air situation.

🎈

Let's circle back to the story from the Introduction about how I used guidance from this handbook to successfully navigate the first major Canadian wildfire smoke event of 2023 with no breathing problems. Keep in mind, I live in upstate New York, much closer to the source of the fires than New York City and Washington, D.C., which received most of the press you may have seen or read.

Here is what my family and I did to protect our home:

1. I checked the air quality on a daily basis with a phone app that also provides the air quality forecast for the next day. In my area, outdoor AQI is typically "green" and in some infrequent instances "yellow." Monday June 5th, I saw that the AQI was forecast as "red" for the following day, so I knew that some sort of serious air quality event was coming. We closed all of the windows in the house, which we generally leave open at this time of year for fresh air—battening down the hatches!

2. Throughout the event, I continued to keep an eye on air quality predictions and measurements from local air quality stations. At one point, the AQI crept all the way up to 460, deep into "maroon" AQI territory!

3. I kept an eye on weather reports throughout the event. The reports clearly indicated a steady wind coming towards our town directly from the northwest (where the Canadian wildfires were located) at 8 miles per hour for the extent of the event. This slow, steady wind was what was able

to carry so much smoke so consistently over our area. It was clear from weather forecasts that the weather patterns would likely change on the fourth day, and shifting winds and/or rain might finally push the rest of the smoke out of our area.

4. During the event we made sure that our plug-in air purifiers with HEPA filtration were on, running on a high setting, and that they had clean filters. We have a plug-in air monitor from a company that makes RESET-accredited indoor air quality monitors.[101] It measures a number of things, including PM2.5 levels. We keep it in the kitchen, which is a relatively central space open to the living room and dining room. I regularly checked its display throughout the event to understand how our indoor air was doing. I could see that even though we had our windows closed, as the air outside got worse, the air quality inside very slowly got worse as well. When it got to a certain point inside, we cranked up our air purifiers to full capacity until the air quality monitor showed that indoor air improved back to a level I was comfortable with.

5. We largely stayed indoors for the event. When I *did* need to leave the house, I wore my N95 mask and traveled with a small HEPA air purifier in my car.

6. We practiced relaxation! We played games and did other fun indoor activities to stay happy and in chill spirits.

Thankfully, as the weather forecast indicated would happen, the weather patterns shifted on the fourth day and things started to clear up.

Of course, we also made mistakes and learned a few things!

---

101 RESET, "Indoor Air Quality Monitors," accessed March 29, 2025, reset.build/directory/monitors/type/indoor.

1. I forgot to fully close a window in the master bedroom closet (for some odd reason our closet has a window). Even this single window being cracked open brought a *ton* of unwanted smoke into the house. The bedroom stank like a campfire.
2. I learned that our house is not good to spend more than three days in with all the windows closed. We do not have a mechanical ventilation system, and so it is essential in our house to have open windows (at least occasionally) to bring in fresh air. I watched the CO_2 levels on our meter go up and up to a level that was a bit higher than what I prefer by the end of the third day. If the event had gone on longer, I would have made plans for us to relocate to an area not affected by the smoke for a few days.

All in all, it was a great success, and we all came out healthy. That's what counts!

To close this handbook, I ask you to stand strong in your Air Self-Care. It's a multifaceted practice and a long game that we can all play to achieve better lives for ourselves, our loved ones, our pets, and our communities.

Good luck and take care!

Love, M

EXERCISE I: Level #2—Air Quality Questionnaire

Items you'll need:

1. A blank piece of paper to write down your answers and a writing utensil of choice.

2. A notebook for anything you learn along the way that you might want to reference in the future, like model numbers of systems in your building, names of companies who can conduct radon testing, follow-up questions you want to look into later, etc.

3. Optional: Anything that makes you feel smart, confident and tenacious, like glasses, a clipboard, a pocket handkerchief and/or a lanyard with some flair.

Air Quality Sleuthing Prompts

#1: Ventilation Systems

Is my building mechanically or naturally ventilated?[102] (If you're not sure, please check out Appendix II: How Do I Know if My Building Has Mechanical Ventilation?)

For buildings with mechanical ventilation

- When was the last time maintenance was conducted?
- How often is maintenance required to be conducted?
- Where is the building's outdoor air intake located?
    - o Is the area clear of debris?
    - o Is the area protected from sources of air contamination like people smoking, cars idling, or major construction close by?

---

102 Note, some buildings include a mix of mechanical and natural ventilation. If this is the case in your building, answer the questions in both sections below and make a note of which parts of the building they pertain to.

- Does my building have a plan for when outside air coming in through the air intake happens to be polluted? (For example, during a wildfire smoke event.) What are the details of this plan?

For buildings with natural ventilation:

- What processes are required to be conducted every day to ensure that the building is correctly naturally ventilated (e.g., opening windows at certain times)?
- Are there any spaces in my building where people spend time that don't have access to regular fresh air? (For example, a frequently used room in the middle of a large building with no windows.) If yes, how can I make these places better ventilated? Or could I move the activities that happen in that space to a location in the building that has good ventilation?

#2: Have the "silent killer" gas risks been addressed at my building?

Carbon monoxide (CO)

- Are there any possible sources of CO in or near my building that I can actively try to prevent?
- Are there working carbon monoxide (CO) detectors in my building?
  - o If no, add them!
  - o If yes:
    - i. When was the last date the batteries were changed?
    - ii. Per the directions that came with the CO detectors, are there enough CO detectors for my building? Are they located and installed correctly? Is there someone who takes care of replacing the batteries and changing the detectors when necessary?

Radon

- Does my building already have a radon mitigation system?
    - o If yes, does it require any regular love and care to keep up the good work?
    - o If no, has anyone checked out if there's a risk of radon at my building?

Natural Gas

- Does my building use natural gas for heating or cooking?
- What is the number to call if you suspect a leak?

#3: How clean is my building?

- Is the building dusty?
- Are any cooking appliances like ovens, stoves, or microwaves dirty? Which ones?
- Are there any leaks, drips, or spots with sitting water? What can I do to fix them?
- Trash, recycling, and compost:
    - a. Is waste taken out of the building before it starts to smell?
    - b. Are there lids on waste bins?
    - c. Are refrigerators cleaned out regularly?

#4: What is the inside of my building cleaned with?

- Are there any bleach-based products used or stored near any ammonia-based products?
- Do any of my cleaning products have inhalation warnings associated with them?
- Do vacuum cleaners used in my building have HEPA filters?

#5: Regarding renovation work:

1. Have any renovations or any type of interior construction been done recently in the building, such as painting,

new cabinets, or new floors? If yes, what? Are there any inhalation warnings associated with the new materials?

2. Have any new pieces of furniture been added recently? If yes, what? Do they have inhalation warnings?

3. If renovations have been done recently, was the nearby ventilation and conditioning equipment in the building protected? (For example, perhaps the ventilation system was shut off and the vents were covered with plastic while a contractor was removing old flooring and installing new flooring.)

#6: Is there a possibility that polluted outdoor air could affect my building?

1. Can I think of anything in my neighborhood that might be polluting the local outdoor air? (You can reference Chapter II: Outdoor Air Basics for ideas.)

2. If yes, are there indications that the building has air leaks such as drafty areas, visible gaps under doors, or sounds when it is windy outside?

3. Does my building use any air filtration? If yes, do the air filters match typical outdoor air pollutants in my area? (For more details on how to match filters to air pollutants, please turn to Chapter VIII: How Do We Fix Air Quality.)

#7: What is the shoe situation?

1. Are there mats or grates for people to clean their shoes on as they pass through the door?

2. Do people take off their shoes when they enter?

#8: Time to interview the folks in the building!

Find at least three people in your building to interview about their experience with the building's air quality. Ask them the following questions (and feel free to ask more if there's something specific to your building that you could use feedback on):

1. Are there any rooms in the building where the air feels stale?

2. Are there any rooms you avoid because you feel a bit drowsy, headachy, or lightheaded when you spend much time in them?

3. If you feel comfortable sharing, do you suffer from asthma, allergies, or other breathing sensitivities?

   o   If yes, do you ever feel symptoms coming on in any areas of the building and then feel better when you leave them?

When interviewing people, you can can either include the actual names of those surveyed or mark each person as anonymous person #1, #2, etc. if anonymity is needed to get honest information you can share.

Overall Findings

Once you've completed the questions above, please take a minute to review your findings and respond to the prompts below:

1. List all possible sources or causes of poor air quality in the building.

2. Name the items to follow up on based on your findings.

EXERCISE II: Level #3—Basic Air Quality Testing

Items you'll need:

- At least one air sensor, as described in Chapter VII: Level #3. Multiple sensors will speed up the process.
- A spreadsheet to keep data logged in. If you're computer averse, you can create a spreadsheet by hand on a large sheet of paper with a straightedge and writing utensil.
- Optional: Anything that makes you feel cool, official, comfortable and sharp, like a water bottle, supportive shoes, fresh cup of coffee, snazzy scarf, or clipboard.

Steps

- Make a list of the following rooms in the building:
  - o Rooms where people and pets spend the most time
  - o Rooms (not already on your list) where you suspect there could potentially be air quality issues based on your previous sleuthing

You can add more rooms than these as you wish. Just keep in mind that each extra room will be an extra time investment. Make sure all of your room labels are very clear—like "sister Sally's bedroom" or "6th floor restroom on NE end of building."

- Decide the length of time you'll use for each air quality measurement. Different types of air quality sensors will take different amounts of time to register a correct reading. Think of it like a thermometer you would use to check on a fever: you need to wait for a period of time until it flashes or beeps to get an accurate temperature. Learn about your sensor and the recommended measurement time. If you can't find any information on your particular sensor, you can choose to take half-day or full-day measurements. (In this case, you set up your sensor, set an alarm for when you'll check back, and then when the alarm goes off you'll take the reading and move the sensor to the next location.)

- Make a plan for which rooms on your list you're going to measure at which times, then measure them and diligently log the data in your spreadsheet. Make sure to note in your spreadsheet the date and time of each test. If you'd like to be a super stellar scientist, I recommend that you also log next to each room:
  o Weather conditions outside
  o AQI outside
  o Whether or not there are windows in that room
  o Whether or not there are ventilation vents in that room
  o Whether doors or windows were open during the test
  o Any other factors you think could affect air quality in that room (like maybe it's got an oven, a kitty litter box, or chemical storage)

It is best if you can take the measurements back to back for the rooms on your list instead of having big gaps between readings. Having more than one sensor will speed up this process. Note: read the directions for your sensor to understand the best place to put it in a room so you can get a good reading. Using the thermometer analogy again, you probably won't get a good reading on your fever if you stick the thermometer under your chin instead of under your tongue. It's the same deal with air sensors. You'll want to put it in a spot where a normal person would be breathing (i.e., about 3–6 ft above the floor) and not right next to a window or ventilation vent where the air quality could be really different than in the rest of the room.

- After you have measured all of the rooms, see if any of the measurements were in a "bad" or a "not great" range for any of the parameters that you were measuring. Many air sensor devices will tell you if levels are "bad" or not by color coding the readings, or by including a guide that you can compare your results to. If you're flying without a guide, you can consult the internet to find WHO (World Health Organization) recommendations.

- Use data to make improvements in any rooms that have "bad" results:
    o Use your developed air quality sleuthing skills to identify Bad $H!T in the room. Remove the Bad $H!T as best you can (check out Chapter VIII: How to Fix Bad Air Quality for ideas).
    o Re-measure spaces that had moderate-to-poor air quality to see if your air quality fix worked. If results are still bad, continue making improvements and re-measuring until you get a result you're happy with. Alternatively, you may decide to throw in the towel and instead turn the space into a closet or another type of room people don't spend a lot of time in.

EXERCISE III: Level #4—Basic DIY Ventilation Assessment

Items You'll Need:

1. A sensor that measures CO_2 (or more than one if you have a large building and want this exercise to go faster).
2. A spreadsheet to keep data logged in.
3. Optional: Anything that makes you feel cool, official, comfortable, and sharp, such as sunglasses, insoles, bubble tea and/or rockabilly blaring in your old-school, faux wood, over-ear headphones.

Steps

1. Make a list of rooms where people and pets usually spend more than 10 minutes a day. You may be able to use your list from Exercise I: Basic Air Quality Testing. Put a special mark next to any room you'd like to take an especially close look at, such as:

   o   Any room that didn't perform well in your Basic Air Quality Testing exercise.

   o   Any room where doing the Use Your Mind assessment from Chapter VI revealed that at least one person believes it is regularly stuffy or they have trouble breathing there.

   o   Any room where good quality air is super important, like rooms where babies, grandparents, or people with breathing sensitivities spend a lot of time.

2. Figure out the best time of day to measure CO_2 levels in each room and mark it in your spreadsheet. Remember, it's best to take readings when people and pets are in the

spaces or right after they leave. Here are some examples of good times to take CO2 readings:

- o Bedrooms—after people wake up and leave in the morning
- o Offices—while people are working midday, or right after people leave at the end of the workday
- o Dining areas—while people are eating or right after they leave

3. Make a plan of which dates and times you'll measure each room and note these in your spreadsheet.

4. Each day you are measuring, first take a reading of the outdoor air CO2 level and enter it into your spreadsheet.

5. Take measurements in all rooms listed in your plan and enter your data into your spreadsheet. Optional but recommended: when you're taking each measurement, include the following notes next to each entry:

- o Are any windows in the space opened or closed?
- o Are any doors to the space opened or closed?
- o How many people and pets are in the space while the sensor is taking its reading?
- o Are there any mechanical ventilation system elements in that room, and are they on? For example, maybe you see a vent bringing air into the room, then you check and see that it is fully open and feel air coming out of it.

6. After you have measured all of the rooms, characterize the ventilation in each space using the table "Ventilation Scoring Based on CO2 Level" that was introduced earlier and is included again below for easy reference, and add the "ventilation rating" into your spreadsheet for each entry.

CO2 Level	Ventilation Rating
Exact same as outside	Awesome
Less than 1,000 ppm	Good
1,000–1,500 ppm	OK
1,500–2,500 ppm	Not great
2,500–5,000 ppm	Bad
>5,000 ppm	Very bad, especially if a person could potentially be in this space for more than 8 hours at a time

7. Identify any rooms that have scored "Not Great," "Poor," or "Very Bad." If you're a crusader for excellent ventilation, you can also identify rooms that only scored "OK."

8. Use data to make improvements in any rooms that had "bad" results in step 7:

   o   Use your air quality sleuthing skills to identify what might be causing any poor situations. Remember, ventilation is when buildings breathe air in and out—so what is preventing air from getting in, getting out, and/or flowing through the space?

   o   After you make any adjustments, re-measure problem spaces to see if the CO2 levels have improved. If results are still "bad," continue making improvements and re-measuring until you get a result you're happy with (or you decide to cry uncle and turn the room into a closet or another type of room people don't spend a lot of time in).

APPENDIX I: FOR THOSE WHO ARE UNSATISFIED WITH THE STATUS QUO

Y ou might get to this point in the book and have questions like:

- Why doesn't my government have adequate laws regarding indoor and outdoor air quality?
- Why doesn't the media cover the dangers of poor air quality as much as wars, COVID-19, and shark attacks?
- Why doesn't the education system cover the basics of how to manage your indoor air quality?
- How can I make a difference?

These are great questions! Here's some places to channel your energy, listed in alphabetical order.

Advocacy Opportunities

Poor air quality doesn't just impact us, our friends, and our families—it also impacts our neighbors, animals, and even plants.

For those out there who like to advocate for protections for the vulnerable, here is a list of vulnerable populations that are especially impacted by poor air quality:

- Children and the elderly, who generally have weaker respiratory systems
- Firefighters, who are regularly exposed to horrible air pollution during fire fighting situations due to highly toxic fumes and other pollutants building materials give off while burning
- Unhoused people, especially those located in highly polluted areas
- People required to live in buildings with no mechanical ventilation, where it is prohibited for safety reasons to open windows for sufficient fresh air. These buildings include certain prisons, homeless shelters, and/or psychiatric wards that may not have the funding or the advocacy to initiate a project to install a robust ventilation solution.
- Economically challenged folks, who often find themselves living in substandard housing in neighborhoods where zoning may not protect them from polluters
- Those with long-term respiratory illness, including asthmatics or folks with long COVID, severe respiratory allergies, etc.
- Workers exposed to significant air pollutants as part of their jobs, like certain factory workers, miners, laundromat workers, nail/hair salon workers, pharma-factory workers, etc.
- The rainforest (which has a very special place in my heart). This ecosystem produces over 20% of the planet's oxygen and absorbs huge amounts of the planet's carbon dioxide (among many other extraordinary things it does!)

There are already groups out there that advocate for clean air—and we could certainly use some more if you have the chutzpah to get something like that off the ground!

Community Building Opportunities

Get a group of like-minded folks together, like a Meetup group, who have a common vision of learning and sharing more about air and air quality. It can be fun to be with other humans, inspire each other, and share ideas! An interesting example of local people banding together is the group GASP (Group Against Smog and Pollution) in Pittsburgh, PA, who serve as a neighborhood watchdog for air pollution.[103] They actively create and run targeted, effective, and also feelgood activities to promote better air quality in their area and engage their community.

Consumer Opportunities

You can show the commercial world that you value good air quality with the way that you spend your money. Here are things that you can do:

- Buy vehicles that create little to no air pollution (including the tires)
- Select cleaning supplies that don't aggravate respiratory sensitivities, especially those of our friends with allergies
- Create demand for air quality technologies that are affordable, accurate, and easy to maintain by taking actions such as purchasing the best options available in your price range and providing detailed customer reviews that will give the company (and future potential purchasers) useful feedback. Such technologies include:

---

103 Group Against Smog & Pollution, accessed March 29, 2025, gasp-pgh.org/.

- o   Air sensor technologies
- o   Air filtration and purification technologies
- o   Ventilation systems
- When purchasing furniture, furnishings, and other "new stuff," select options that specifically don't aggravate respiratory sensitivities, especially those of children and asthmatics.
- Buy used (vintage, antique, secondhand, etc.)

Educational Opportunities

- Advocate at school board meetings that basic air education be included in the curriculum.
- Contact local science teachers and advocate that they include a unit on basic air quality.
- Offer classes in your area on air quality basics.
- Start putting flags outside your building that match the color of the day's outdoor air AQI, as recommended by AirNow.[104]
- Celebrate Air Quality Awareness Week at the beginning of May by holding a community educational event or an *excellent* party.

Legal Opportunities

- Learn about your local air quality protections.
- Find out how your local and national political system works and engage with a goal to get better air quality protections put in place.
- Support groups that are already out there making a difference on the political and legal stage, such as:
  - o   Clean Air Council: charitynavigator.org/ein/231683461

---

104 Air Quality Flag Program, accessed Sept. 17, 2025, airnow.gov/air-quality-flag-program.

o   Earth Justice (lawyers advocating for clean air): earthjustice.org/advocacy-campaigns/clean-air
- Learn about previous legal successes, such as:
    o   US Clean Air Act: epa.gov/clean-air-act-overview/clean-air-act-requirements-and-history
    o   UK Clean Air Act: navigator.health.org.uk/theme/clean-air-act-1956#:~:text=The%20Clean%20Air%20Act%20of,of%20coal%20and%20industrial%20activities.

Media Opportunities

- Contact your local media stations to request more content on air quality.
- Hold rockin' air quality-related events and invite the media to attend.
- Post about air quality events, air quality news, and air quality facts across social media platforms.

Research and Development (R&D) Opportunities

- Support R&D efforts related to air sensors, air filtration, and air purification.
- Support R&D efforts related to cost-effective methods of "scrubbing" air for:
    o   Power plants
    o   Factories
    o   Vehicles
    o   Air/space travel
- Support R&D efforts related to developing products with reduced air quality impact, especially in the following industries:

- o Beauty products
- o Cleaning products
- o Construction products
- o Furniture
- o Fertilizer and pesticide products

Really: the sky's the limit here. These ideas are just ideas to get you going. Be creative and don't get discouraged!

APPENDIX II: HOW DO I KNOW IF MY BUILDING HAS MECHANICAL VENTILATION?

*I*t's not always initially clear whether or not a building has mechanical ventilation. Here is guidance to help you figure it out.

First, a mechanically ventilated building will usually have some (and probably all!) of the elements below:

- A spot where outdoor air is sucked into the building by mechanical equipment, called the **outdoor air intake**. This is often on a rooftop or in another spot high above the ground, far away from polluters like vehicles driving by and people smoking on the sidewalk. Outdoor air intakes can take many different forms, so you may need to do some research on different pieces of equipment and vents you find at your building to know if you've found one. Below is an example of an outdoor air intake on a building rooftop:

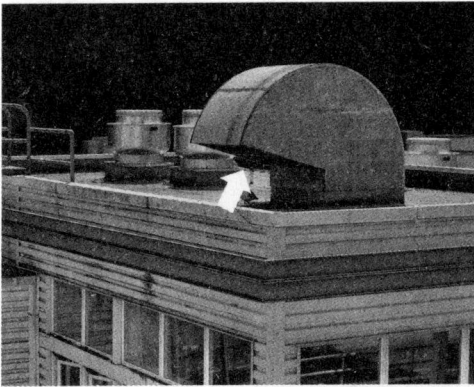

An outdoor air intake located on a rooftop. Air from above the building (i.e., above the level of car exhaust and other typical street level air pollutants) enters in through the large hole indicated by the arrow, travels through the building's ductwork, and then enters into rooms for people and pets to breathe. Photo credit: Isaac Gallinati

- **Ducts** that carry air to different parts of the building. Some ducts are silver metal, some are painted to be the same color as a ceiling, and some are even made of colored industrial cloth. The key is that they move air around the building.

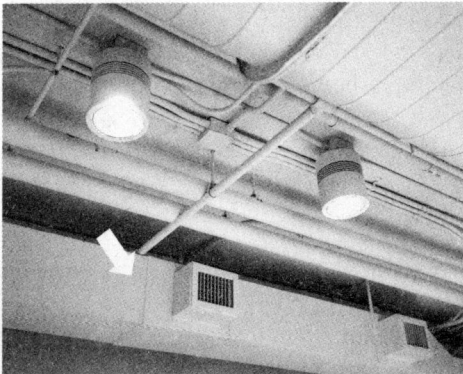

The arrow points to an overhead metal duct carrying air into a room. The grates on the side are where air exits the ductwork. Photo credit: Drew Beamer (arrow added)

- **Vents** that either provide air or suck it out of a room. These can be on ceilings, walls or even floors.

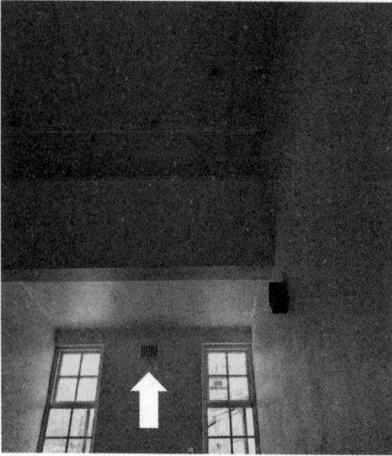

The added arrow in the image to the left points to the grate where air enters the room from ductwork behind the wall. Ductwork is often located behind walls and inside ceilings. Photo credit: Johan Matthee

- A **"mechanical room"** or **"equipment room"** that includes equipment that has air ducts connected to it (not just a room with water pipes and electrical panels).

Now, it is common in homes and some other types of buildings to have systems that move air around that are *not part of a ventilation system that exchanges new fresh air from outside with old indoor air.* **Alert:** If your building only has one of the systems described below (exhaust fans and conditioning systems), your building does not necessarily have a complete mechanical ventilation system.

Exhaust Fans

These are typically found in the bathroom or in the kitchen. These systems will take dirty air from the room they are in and dump it outside of your building. They do not bring any fresh air into your building like a human body's respiratory system would. Instead, these systems are analogous to a human body's "burping" and "tooting" mechanisms that allow contaminated air out in short spurts when needed.

Conditioning Systems

These are systems that move air around with the sole goal of changing its temperature. While some buildings have mechanical ventilation systems *and* conditioning systems, many buildings *only* have conditioning systems. Conditioning systems are like your body's very important thermoregulation system,[105] which is made up of the circulatory system, sweat glands, skin, and parts of the brain that keep the body heated and cooled. The body's thermoregulation system notedly does *not* include the respiratory system.

The way you can tell that a building only has a conditioning system and *not* a ventilation system is whether or not there is an outdoor air intake. A ventilation system *must* have an outdoor air intake, whereas a conditioning system will not have one.

It is actually quite common practice in the construction of houses and building projects with a tight budget to provide a conditioning system and no mechanical ventilation system. Some of these buildings will have a central heating system or central air conditioning (cooling) system that has similar elements that you'd see in a mechanical ventilation system, like ducts and vents, but there's no mechanical ventilation actually happening! These systems are just moving around heated or cooled indoor air for temperature control.

105 Zia Sherrell, "What is thermoregulation, and how does it work?", *MedicalNewsToday*, October 8, 2021, medicalnewstoday.com/articles/thermoregulation.

For example, it is common to install a "split system," where a big square piece of equipment is placed outside the building that has hot air blowing out of it. Then, inside the building, ducts carry cooled air that blows out of vents into the rooms. Is there mechanical ventilation happening with this system? Let's take a closer look!

This type of system operates very similarly to a window air conditioning (AC) unit. Below is a simple diagram that shows how a window AC works. For some context, in this diagram, we're looking at the window AC from the side: the split in the middle is the window it sits in, the black arrow on the far left side is the vent that blows cool air into the building, and the grille on the far right side is what you would see blowing hot air outside of the building.

AIR CONDITIONING SYSTEM

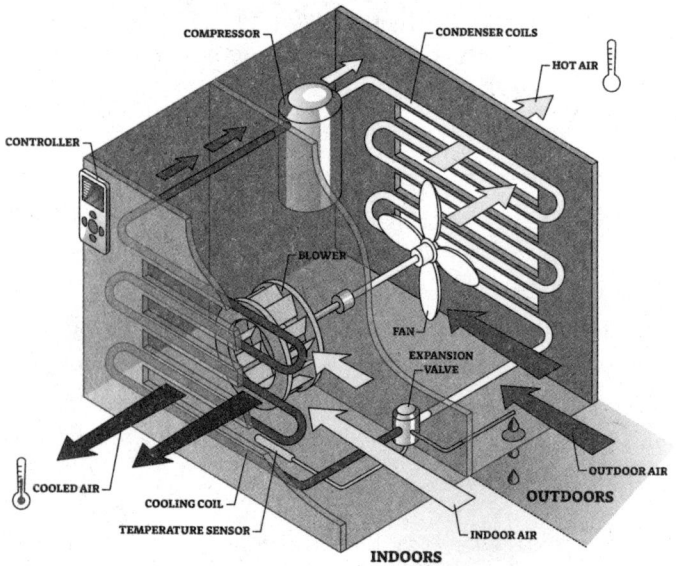

Now, first check out the loop that runs around the entire piece of equipment with coils near both the front and back vents. This loop contains a **refrigerant** that picks up heat from inside the building (in the dark coil) and drops off the heat when it travels outside the building (in the white coil).

Next, check out the two completely separate paths that air takes through the window AC.

Air Path #1—Inside	Air Path #2—Outside
1. Warm air from inside the building is sucked into the indoor part of the unit	1. Air from outside the building is sucked into the outdoor part of the unit
2. The air passes over the cool (dark) refrigerant coils	2. The air passes over the hot (white) refrigerant coils
3. The refrigerant coils suck the heat out of the air, resulting in cooled air	3. The refrigerant coils dump their extra heat into the air, resulting in heated air
4 The cooled air is blown out of the vent right back into the building	4. The heated air is blown out of the vent, back to the outdoors where it came from

You see that zero air actually crosses from the outside to the inside of the building or vice versa! This means that *zero ventilation* is happening. Your refrigerator uses a similar system, which is why the back is warm. As we know from KipKip's tale, refrigerators do *not* have ventilation.

As mentioned before, many homes are air conditioned (cooled) by split systems that operate similarly to this window AC, only the parts look different. They have a similar loop, with refrigerant that passes heat from the inside to the outside of the building and two air paths that don't cross.

Again, these systems may have ducts to carry air that has recently been heated or cooled around the house into different rooms and vents that the air comes out of. Just remember, if there is no outdoor air intake (that brings air from outside *into* the building), the building has no mechanical ventilation.

If you're still stumped on whether or not your building has a mechanical ventilation system, you can call a local building systems professional to come out and take a look!

APPENDIX III: AIR QUALITY INDEX 101

*H*ow is AQI (air quality index) calculated? Here is the process:

1. Major air pollutants are measured in testing stations across the globe.
2. These measurements are converted into standardized AQI values. Try AirNow's online AQI calculator.
3. Whichever major pollutant AQI value is the highest at any given time is listed as the "overall AQI" value.

This AQI value is then posted, and typically the website it's posted on will also tell you the name of the naughty pollutant that has set the overall number.

For example, let's say measurements were taken of the following four major pollutants, and the AQI values for each were calculated as follows:

- PM2.5—AQI value 85
- PM10—AQI value 15
- O3 (ozone)—AQI value 95

- SO2 (sulfur dioxide)—AQI value 12

In this case, the overall AQI value will be listed as 95. When you check the AQI in that area, it would say 95, ozone (since the high ozone value is what sets the overall AQI value.)

SPECIAL THANKS

T'd like to first thank my Uncle Mark for sparking enough Scandinavian-Midwesterner bravado and can-do attitude in me to put together the first sketch of this book. I'd like to then thank my brother Preston for supporting me through early obstacles as I started to realize how much work it is to *actually* take on writing a book.

A big thanks to Uncle James, Aunt Jan, friend San, friend Damian, sister Windsor, and dear Andy for taking the time to read and candidly comment on my first completed draft of the book, and asking questions that led me down many new exciting rabbit holes. A hearty thanks to Meghan for being a highly detailed and frank early editor, a killer with dreaded citation formatting, and a warm-hearted cheerleader as I wrapped up edits for the publisher.

A huge thanks to the Microcosm team. I am still astounded that I found a publisher that was such a good match for how I wanted to present my work to the world. Everyone on their team that I've met and worked with has been incredibly intelligent, thoughtful, curious, good humored, and quite lovely. Also, they treat their writers like divas, which has really tickled my funny bone throughout the entire process. Buy their books! We need more folks like them in business.

Thanks to those who have inspired my interest in all things air throughout my life. Special call-out to my vocal coach, opera singer David Reck, who significantly helped me strengthen my respiratory system.

A big thank you to everyone in the world who has been paying attention to air (while most of us forget about it) and who have been fighting to keep our planet's air in the best breathing condition possible.

A big hug and a kiss to dear Andy who has supported me from the beginning to the end of this process, and never had a doubt that I could get to the end of the road. Also, much gratitude to the cats that have kept me company during long hours of writing, especially Diggory.

Finally—I'm thankful that this process has transformed me from an "expert in air" to knowing I've really *just* scratched the surface of everything there is to know about the air I live in. Around every new corner, worlds have opened up!

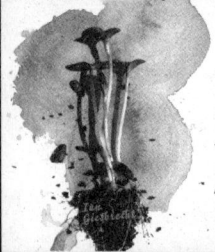
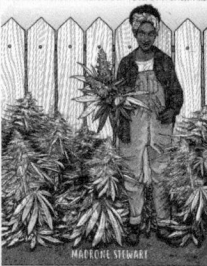
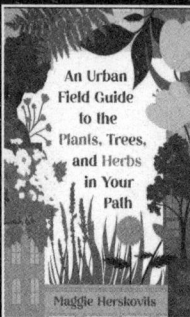
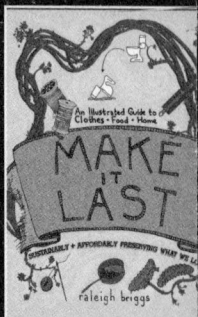
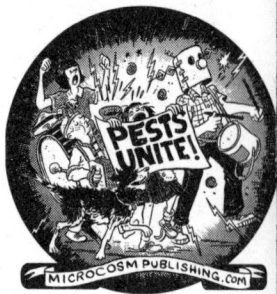
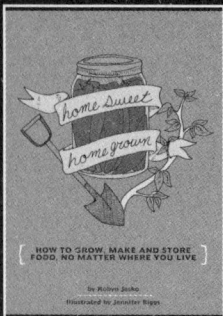
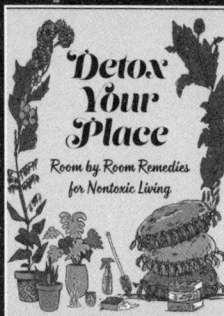
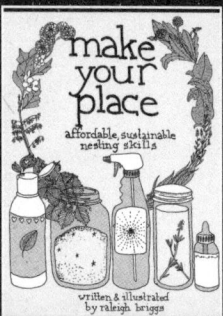
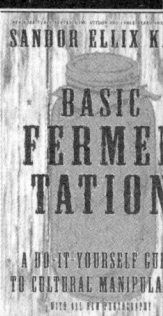